PALEO ITALIAN
Cooking

AUTHENTIC ITALIAN
GLUTEN-FREE FAMILY RECIPES

CINDY BARBIERI

Forewords by **ROBB WOLF** and **BOBBY SOPER**
Photography by **NICOLE ALEKSON**

TUTTLE Publishing

Tokyo | Rutland, Vermont | Singapore

CONTENTS ⚜⚜⚜⚜⚜⚜⚜⚜⚜⚜⚜⚜⚜⚜⚜

Foreword by Robb Wolf

New York Times Bestselling Author of
The Paleo Solution

When I think about Italians and traditions, Cindy Barbieri stands out as a champion of the joyful practice of gathering around the table to eat, laugh and share stories of the day with family and friends. Everyone fortunate enough to enjoy Cindy's hospitality leaves with a dish or a gift to take home as a thank-you for spending time with her. She enjoys all aspects of entertaining, but most of all she loves cooking for her guests.

Cindy's family is from Italy, and she visits Tuscany every year. Upon returning home to Massachusetts, she recreates Italian dishes inspired by meals enjoyed on picturesque mountaintops overlooking the vineyards of central Italy. Since becoming part of the Paleo community, Cindy has been transforming traditional dishes, along with new inspirations, into authentic Paleo Italian recipes. Her crowd-pleasing Tuscan twist adds something new to the Paleo world, including popular and flavorful one-pot recipes that are suitable for both weeknight family dining and entertaining.

This cookbook will show you how to make restaurant-quality Paleo Italian recipes right in your own kitchen!

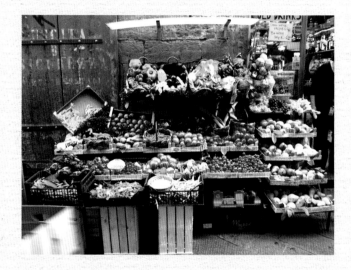

Foreword by Bobby Soper

President & CEO, *Mohegan Sun*

When you spend time with Cindy Barbieri, the word "passion" comes to mind. Whether it's her passion for sharing her culinary creations with the world; or her passion for helping others who are less fortunate via her efforts with Foodshare; or her passion for showcasing her talents through her *Cindy's Table* magazine and this cookbook, her energy emanates from everything she does. This energy is contagious and uplifting. We are proud to be associated with such a talented individual who creates smiles on the faces of all her viewers, readers, and people in the community who she has helped.

ABOUT CINDY

Cindy's love for food began before she could reach the counter in her Nana's Italian kitchen. Her grandmother Nicolina, who was from Naples, loved to be surrounded by her family. She could always be found in the kitchen stirring a large pot of sauce or making lasagna to feed the neighborhood. Cindy is a lot like her Nana, as she enjoys sharing her love for cooking and preparing her family's favorite meals when all the kids are home visiting.

Every meal has a story of Cindy and Nana in the kitchen together, and Cindy's eyes sparkle when these tales are shared with family and friends. Cindy's two sisters also love to reminisce about their childhood. Although the sisters sometimes disagree about the way Nana made certain recipes, they always have fun when they get a chance to cook together—with, of course, a glass of wine in hand.

Cindy's infectious enthusiasm for Italian food pervades all of her recipes, which demonstrate the passion inspired by her Italian heritage and her extensive travels throughout Italy. Her Italian style of cooking is flavorful yet clean, and very approachable. The recipes are not complicated, and many of them can be made in advance, but they'll always be the star of the party!

Cindy and her husband Glenn love to entertain in their large country home in Marlborough, Connecticut. Most of the recipes in this book appear regularly in Cindy's kitchen—especially her antipasti, which is always offered to family and friends. Other favorites are the spinach and artichoke rolls and her delicious frittatas. She always serves Italian chopped salad alongside Tuscan favorites such as anchovy pizza or Roman braised eggplant. A pot of sauce or meatball and kale soup will be simmering on the stove on the weekends. On any given night at Cindy's, you might be served her chicken scaloppine in a caper sauce or even osso buco; if she feels like seafood, you could have the salmon with lemon, capers and thyme. Cindy's desserts are light and easy, but very Italian. This book offers a unique take on the flavors of Tuscany. Cindy's hope in sharing these homemade Tuscan Paleo recipes is that you will feel like part of her family and share her love for the taste of Italy.

BUON APPETITO!

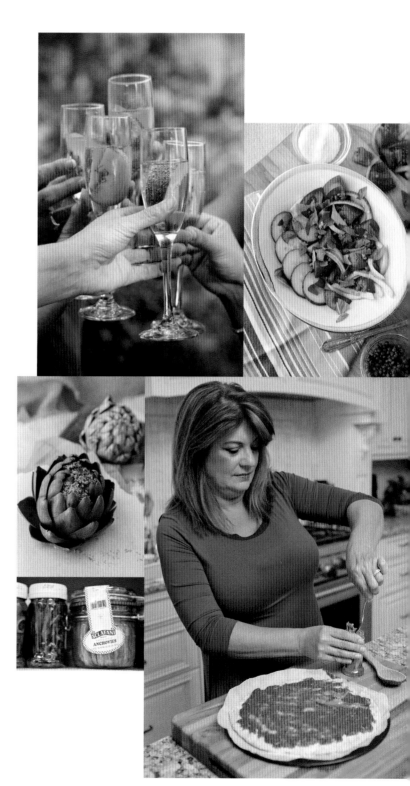

WELCOME TO MY WORLD

am so happy you are here to share what I love most: cooking for my family and friends while drinking wine in my kitchen! I've found that inviting new friends home to share one of my homemade Paleo Italian dishes with a glass of wine is a wonderful way to deepen a friendship.

My family is from Naples, Italy, and many of the Paleo Italian recipes in this book are based on my family traditions and the flavors from this area. My husband and I also spend two weeks in Italy every year. We especially love the Tuscan area of central Italy, with its natural cobbled streets, wide-open windows, and friendly folks standing outside ready to welcome you into their restaurants or shops; but there are countless beautiful parts of Italy to be discovered while traveling through the countryside. I've been lucky enough to have traveled throughout Europe and the U.S., and I have found that I feel most at home in Italy. The importance of food and family in everyday life really resonates with my values.

Having spent a lot of time in my grandmother's kitchen growing up, I'm thrilled to have this opportunity to share my extraordinary and easy cooking, which represents my heritage and my love for good, healthy food. In this book, I've included dishes I serve to my family and friends, many of which represent dishes my grandmother, Nana, made for us. My best childhood memories are of gatherings for birthdays, graduations, weddings, Sunday dinners or simple get-to-

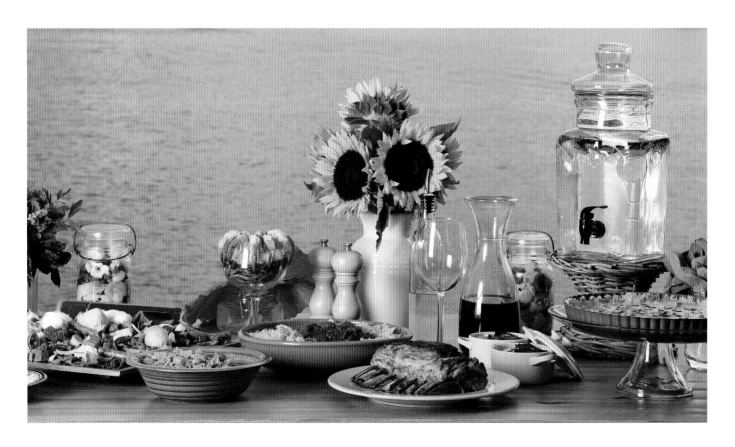

gethers—in which every conversation either began or ended with food. Nana had a very easygoing approach to life: always have enough food to feed the entire family and whoever stops by. Being old-fashioned, she also told me that the way to a man's heart is through his stomach. "Feed your man," she said, "and he'll always come home to you." My approach to cooking is very similar to my grandmother's—keep it simple and add lots of flavor using fresh herbs! The quality of the ingredients plays a very important part in any recipe and enhances the beauty of each dish.

I love easy, authentic Italian food that can be prepared in advance without a lot of mess, and which are equally suitable for weeknight dinners or special occasions.

A typical Italian dinner is served family-style, with wine and laughter.

Weekends often involve more of a multicourse extravaganza that may last a few hours. Because I'm a bit of a selfish mother, it makes me happy to have my family at the table for a few uninterrupted hours, all of us enjoying delicious food together. In this book, I will show you how much fun cooking at home truly is, and how it offers quality time with the people you love around you. In Italy, families spend hours together eating several small meals and drinking local wine. There's no need to consume a large plate of food in a single sitting; eating Italian-style means making a meal into more of an event, taking your time, with the food enhancing the special moments you spend together.

When I decided to leave corporate America and follow my passion into the kitchen, it was a very natural transition. I'm able to make great food for my family and friends every day. I feel blessed to have this opportunity to share my family traditions as well as all of the new recipes coming from my kitchen. I also deeply appreciate my husband's willingness to make time for us to travel throughout Italy each year and enjoy the amazing food, views and wine. These trips have inspired me to create great food using all natural ingredients, and to embrace my Italian heritage. It's a great pleasure to share my travels to Italy, my family traditions and authentic Italian recipes with you, and I hope you enjoy the results.

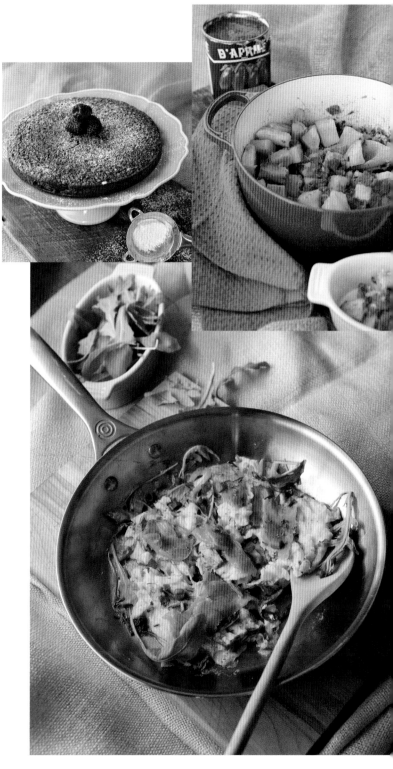

Top left: Chocolate Almond Torte (page 157)
Top right: Venetian Potatoes (page 140)
Above: Scrambled Eggs with Smoked Salmon & Arugula (page 52)

THE PALEO ITALIAN LIFESTYLE

This cookbook assumes that you have some familiarity with the Paleo lifestyle and you're ready to take your skills up a notch to create authentic Italian recipes for your family or friends. If you're new to Paleo, there are many books and online resources that offer a sound introduction. The basic principles of Paleo living involve avoiding dairy, grains, legumes, vegetable oils, processed sugar and most other processed foods. I use grass-fed meats and organic vegetables and fruits whenever possible, and I always keep coconut oil, olive oil, nuts and seeds on hand. Paleo and gluten-free diets are not identical, but if you're avoiding gluten, the Paleo lifestyle is a great way to stay healthy.

Back when I was a kid, food was different: my grandfather had a garden and chickens, and most of our food was unprocessed. In today's world, we need to pay attention to everything that goes into our bodies. Eating wholesome food will enhance your life. When I first learned about Paleo, I loved the community's shared enthusiasm for the lifestyle and for longevity. If you want to live a long life and share your history with your children and grandchildren, why not start now? You'll see the difference after making a few small changes, and you'll want to share it with everyone you know.

I've taken the dishes my Nana made for our family and transformed her recipes to fit a Paleo lifestyle. If you're following this path, you may wonder how to incorporate Italian cooking without it being complicated or losing authenticity. In my opinion, coming from deep-rooted Italian family that ate a lot of lamb, veal, poultry and tons of meatballs, it's easy

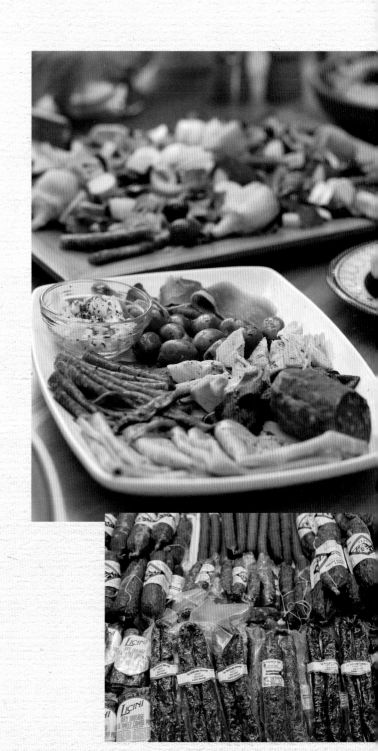

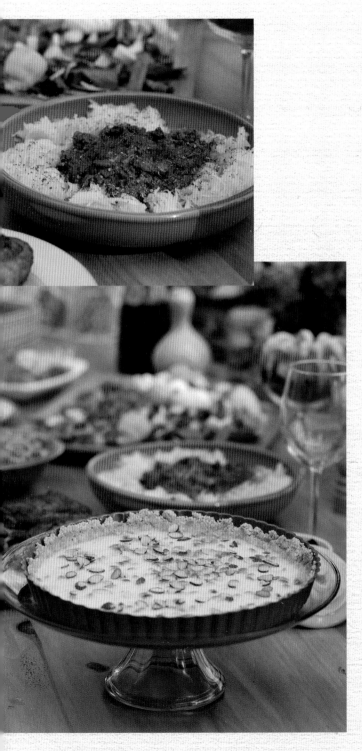

and welcoming. My family and friends all understand my love for cooking, since I prepare enough to feed the neighborhood and welcome company, but they also know I'm cooking Paleo-style. The best part of this transition is that everyone wants to be in the kitchen with me, helping me out. They don't realize it, but I'm teaching them how to cook healthy and keep it easy.

Maybe you're wondering how an Italian can go without pasta, pizza and bread dipped in a big pot of sauce. Well, to be honest, sometimes I don't! Some might call this "cheating," but I call it portion control and making the right choices. Sometimes my Italian nature craves a small bowl of pasta, so I'll indulge it. I am a Paleo advocate, but I also love food and cooking for my family and friends. I feel that if you decide you want that bowl of pasta or slice of pizza, then enjoy it, but don't over-indulge or make a habit of it.

In the course of writing this book over the past four years, I have been updating my Paleo blog and living the Paleo lifestyle. I'm living proof that it's easy to keep your traditions and adhere to the Paleo lifestyle while bringing happiness and love to your guests. I hope that this book creates a place in your heart for my tradition and culture by letting you try out Italian recipes for your friends and family. I also hope to inspire you to create your own traditions for passing on your love and joy through cooking. This book is filled with real food that real people want to eat!

KEEP GOING, AND ENJOY YOUR JOURNEY INTO PALEO ITALIAN CUISINE.

Top: Spaghetti Squash Puttanesca (page 122)
Above: Custard Pie with Pine Nuts & Almonds (page 145)
Opposite top: Italian Chopped Salad (page 45) and
  Antipasto Platter (page 36)
Left: Different types of Italian sausage

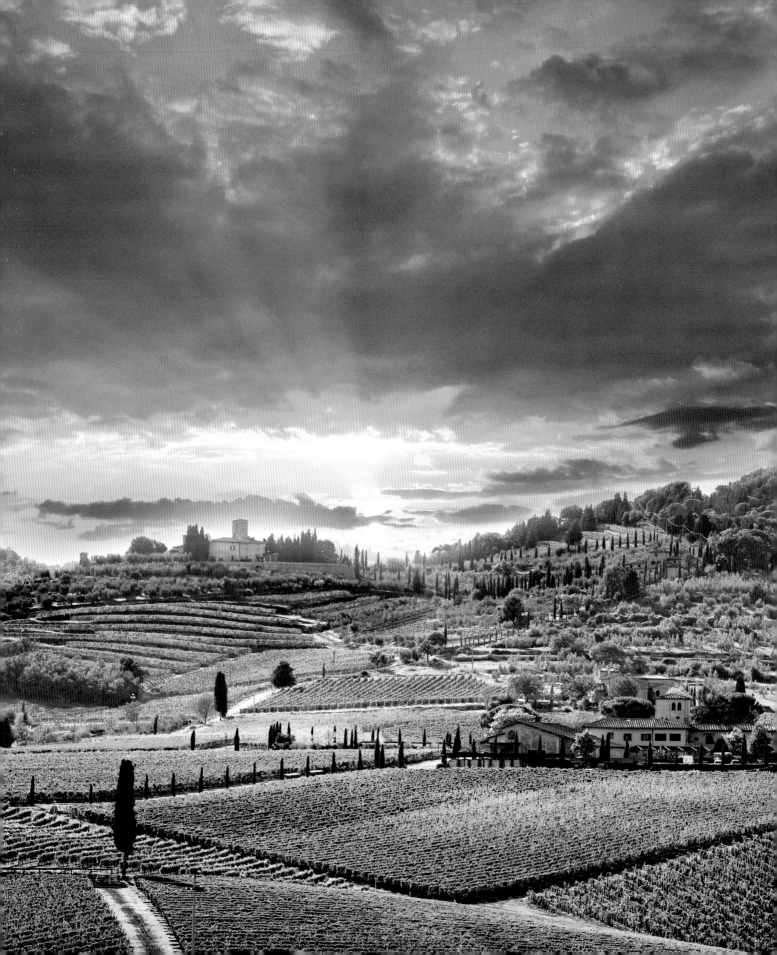

THE SEASONS AND SAVORS OF ITALY

The weather in Italy can vary greatly. The seasons tend to be similar to New England's: summers can be brutally hot and winters can be freezing. When deciding on the best season to choose for a trip to Italy, there are many factors to take into consideration.

Spring in Italy is very beautiful and peaceful. Although early spring may still be a bit chilly, late spring brings warm weather and beautiful flowers. You can enjoy eating outside, and you might even get some swimming in. Traveling to Italy is cheaper in spring than in summer, and far less crowded. There are a number of festive occasions to enjoy; Holy Week festivals take place around Easter, and there are many festivals of light and flowers to celebrate as well. Bring light clothes for hot weather, as well as some sweaters and jackets in case it gets cold. You should also bring a rain jacket and boots, as spring in Italy can be rainy.

Summer is the most popular time for visiting Italy. Many families take their vacations in the summer and want to travel when the weather is nice. Although summer in Italy can be hot and crowded, it's a great time to take advantage of Italy's beautiful beaches and explore its gorgeous cities and medieval villages. Pack light clothes; Italian summers often reach over 100°F (42°C). Definitely bring a bathing suit so you can cool off after a hot summer day!

Another great season for traveling to Italy is fall. The weather is starting to cool off then, but it's still warm enough to enjoy great outdoor activities. It's an ideal time for hiking the mountains or cycling your way through the cities and towns, enjoying the gorgeous fall foliage and natural beauty before winter comes. It's also the best time to taste Italian food, as fresh mushrooms, truffles, olives, and wine are at their peak. There are many food festivals during the fall where you can enjoy delicious Italian treats. As in spring, airfare in fall is usually very cheap, and the enormous summer crowds are gone. Be sure to bring warm clothes—maybe even a winter jacket if you're traveling late in the season. Don't forget your rain jacket, rain boots, and umbrella, too, because November is the rainiest month in Italy. Bring comfortable sneakers for hiking or exploring!

You can always visit Italy in the winter, too. Though it may be cold outside, you can still have a great time, especially if you enjoy winter sports such as skiing or snowboarding. Italy's majestic mountains are a great place for this. The winter holidays in Italy—Christmas, New Year's, and Carnival celebrations, among others—offer an excellent way to witness Italian traditions and sample delicious holiday foods. It's also a great time to explore cultural opportunities such as operas and theater events. Italian winters are beautiful and romantic, with gorgeous snow-covered hills offering amazing views. Be sure to bring plenty of warm clothes with you, including a jacket, gloves, a hat, boots, and scarves.

No matter what the season, the rich culture, beauty and delicious food of Italy never disappoint. In deciding when you want to travel there, consider the kinds of activities you enjoy and factor that into your decision. Spring and fall are great for hiking, summer is great for swimming, and the winter is great for snow sports. Visiting at a time when you can take advantage of your favorite activities will help you make the most out of your Italian vacation.

MY FAVORITE PLACES IN TUSCANY

If you go to Italy, Tuscany is a must-see spot. Located in central Italy, it comprises beautiful countryside, gorgeous hills, the sea coast, and even some islands. It's rich with culture, history, delicious food, and abundant beauty.

Florence, the capital of the region, was home to many influential Western artists and thinkers, including Leonardo da Vinci, Petrarch, Dante, Lorenzo de Medici, Alberti, Bot-

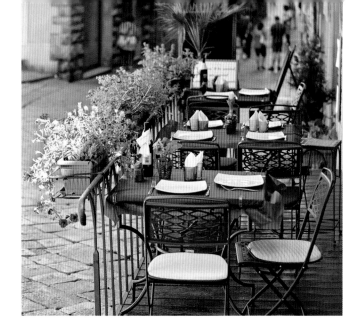

ticelli, and Machiavelli; Tuscany boasts numerous museums dedicated to these important figures. The area also has an abundance of fine art and architecture from the Etruscans, Romans, and the artists and artisans of the Renaissance, with thousands of amazing sculptures, frescoes and architectural masterpieces to enjoy. If you are interested in Tuscany's amazing art and history, I recommend visiting the Leonardo da Vinci Museum in Florence, the Accademia Gallery in Florence, the Siena Cathedral in Siena, the Leaning Tower of Pisa, and the churches of Saint Augustine and San Biagio in Montepulciano, among others.

The foods of Tuscany are justifiably famous. People from all over the world travel there to enjoy fresh homemade pastas, outstanding wines, and delectable pastries. One excellent place to taste the one-of-a-kind Tuscan food is Gigi Trattoria in Lucca, Italy. This quaint Italian restaurant, located on the Piazza del Carmine, has been open since the 1950s, and is well known both for its traditional dishes based on Tuscan cuisine and its friendly service. Another great spot is Osteria del Borgo in Montepulciano, which serves various Tuscan specialties including homemade pasta. It offers indoor and outdoor seating, and when the weather is good, the seats on the terrace offer a stunning view of the Tuscan Hills of the Orcia Valley. Montepulciano is also famous for its fabulous red wines. Be sure to try Nobile di Montepulciano, which is one of the most highly regarded Italian reds.

There are many spectacular places in Tuscany to relax and have fun during your stay. The Castello di Spaltenna, located in Gaiole Chianti, is a magnificent hotel with a castle-like appearance and luxurious rooms appointed in beautiful Tuscan style. The hotel offers all the usual amenities such as Wi-Fi and satellite TV, and also boasts two swimming pools, a gym with sauna and steam room, a tennis court, mountain bikes, a restaurant, and even a boutique. Nearby attractions include the Parish Church of Spaltenna, Vertine Castle, Brolio Castle, Le Miccine winery, Meleto Castle, and Coltibuono Abbey. The Hotel Cala del Porto, located in Punta Ala, right near the Bay of Follonica, is also highly recommended. This five-star seaside resort and hotel offers magnificent views of the water, along with amenities to meet every possible need. You can spend your time here relaxing by going to the spa, lounging in the pool, soaking in the hot tub, or enjoying the hotel's private beach. Activities such as windsurfing, horseback riding, tennis, snorkeling, mini-biking, cycling, golf, mini-golf, and tours of the area are also available. There are many great places to explore in Punta Ala, including Bagno Punta Hidalgo, Bagno Belmare, and Stabilimento Balneare (seaside resort) La Vela.

I know visiting Tuscany can be overwhelming because there are so many tempting places to visit! I hope these suggestions will give you a start on exploring the magnificent culture, history, food, and beauty that this special region of Italy has to offer.

TRADITIONAL DINING IN ITALY

Food is an essential part of Italian life. There are cafés and restaurants everywhere, and if you visit any Italian home, you'll be offered a drink or something to eat before you can even sit down.

There are several regions in Italy—Tuscany being one—each with its own specialties and particular ways of preparing standard dishes. For example, you might order a pasta dish in one region, then order the same dish in another region and find that they are prepared very differently, despite having the same name.

The Italian approach to food is different from what is generally found in America. For example, Italian breakfasts are small, just an accompaniment for morning coffee and talk about the upcoming day. Lunches involve a little more food—a salad and a pizza, for instance. Not a large American-style pizza, though; Italian pizzas are very thin and much smaller, and you won't find them overburdened with toppings or cheese. As a matter of fact, my favorite pizza in Tuscany is simply topped with anchovies, capers and a light sauce with no cheese—just enough to satisfy the midday appetite. Dinner is served later in the evening; many restaurants in Italy don't open until 7:30 p.m. You may walk by a restaurant at 7 p.m. and notice the proprietor's family eating together at a table—they will not open until they are finished with their evening meal.

There is a famous saying in Italy for dinner: "How many courses can you eat?" The first course is the *antipasto*, or appetizer course, which usually consists of olives, cheeses, anchovies, pickled vegetables, and a variety of delicious meats. The next course is the *primi piatto* (first dish), generally consisting of fresh homemade Italian pasta or rice. Next comes the main course, or *secondi piatto*. This is usually made up of meat and a vegetable platter called the *contorno*. Most places serve delectable cuts of meat accom-panied by perfectly cooked fresh vegetables. (If you get a chance, try eating boar—many restaurants serve it, and it is astoundingly good.) The final course is the *dolce*, or sweets. Italian desserts, which are justifiably famous, consist of many pastries, cakes, and other original specialties.

None of these courses are large; in Italy, a course consists of a small plate of food. For example; if you order ravioli, you might get one large piece of ravioli, not a full plate of pasta. When ordering, always remember to give your server all your course selections at once.

Italian restaurants tend to be much more relaxed than restaurants in the U.S. You are never rushed, and servers treat you more like family than a customer. There is a great feeling of closeness among the guests, and it's very easy to make great conversations and find new friends. Some restaurants even have long tables where many customers sit together. I love these types of restaurants, because they allow me to meet many new and interesting people as we bond over delicious Italian food.

While dining in Tuscany, you'll notice that bread is not automatically brought to your table; you have to ask for it. Tuscan bread is not salted, and it's very dense. Be sure to try some before you order, as it may be different from what you're expecting. As for wine, I recommend asking for the house wine in Tuscany. It comes in an unlabeled bottle and it's not expensive, but it is delicious. You may even order a second glass!

If you have a chance to visit Italy, you will treasure your dining experiences. The amazing food, relaxing atmosphere, and friendships that Italian restaurants offer are unique to that country. There are so many wonderful restaurants with great food that it can be hard to choose which one to visit. They each have something unique to offer their guests. I suggest trying as many different Italian restaurants as possible to make the most of the Italian dining experience.

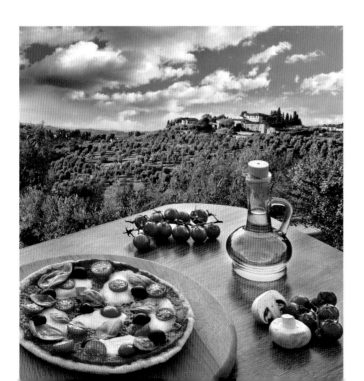

ABOUT THE PALEO LIFESTYLE

As noted previously, this book assumes that you are familiar with the Paleo lifestyle. Whether you're already following the Paleo diet, are living gluten free, or just want to eat healthier, I hope this book helps you make authentic Italian dishes you and your family will enjoy. Your decision to eat better is a great start! You're probably already familiar with the large number of cookbooks, food blogs and other information available about the Paleo lifestyle. Be sure to visit my blog at *CindysTable.com*. I'm not a nutritionist, just a woman who has been cooking since I could reach my Nana's kitchen counter—but I hope my experiences give you more ideas that will help you stay on track.

We all love Italian food, and I hear complaints that you can't enjoy Italian food if you're following the Paleo diet. That's just not true! I have found it easy to do, and often making a recipe Paleo-friendly makes it taste even better.

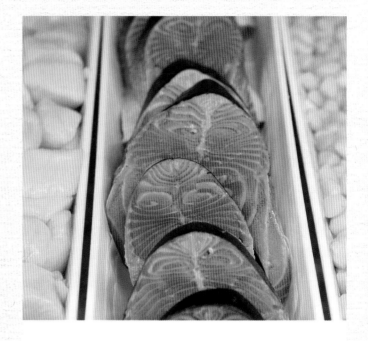

AT THE GROCERY STORE

You have the recipes for the week and your list is made! Make sure you're not hungry when you go shopping. If necessary, make a quick smoothie before you leave. As you shop, follow your list, and don't stray from it unless you find high-priced items like seafood or nut butters that are on sale. Avoid the center aisles with all of the junk food—remember that you're preparing to create wonderful Paleo Italian fare. Also, don't stop at the endcaps, as tempting as they may be. The vendor pays for that endcap, and their goal is to get you to purchase their product and look no further! The same items will be available in the aisle, and you may find another brand there that's less expensive. Have fun while you're shopping; let your imagination run away with you while you consider the incredible healthful meals you're about to create.

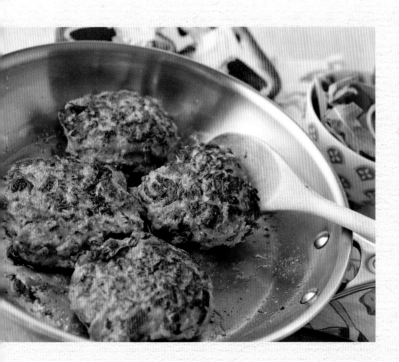

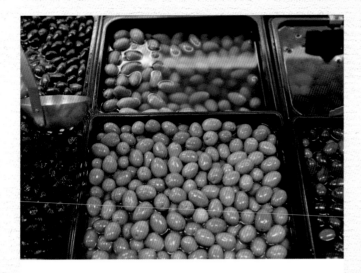

IT STARTS WITH A PLAN

All you need to succeed with Paleo or any other diet is commitment and planning. It's really that simple. I was a single mother for over ten years, and I always served my kids healthy meals. I would sit down and go through the advertisements every Sunday morning, and we would have a "family meeting" to decide what we wanted to eat in the coming week. Then I would drive around to the various markets and gather my ingredients. Now I can go to one or two markets, or even the farmers' market alone, and get what we need. Even though my kids are now grown and have left the house, I still plan the week's meals in advance. The first thing to consider when planning your meals is what's in season. Then review recipes—whether in this cookbook, other cookbooks or online sources—for those main ingredients and make a list of other items you'll need. Before you shop, do an inventory of your pantry, refrigerator and freezer and see what you have on hand, so you won't buy food you don't need. Then go online and find out what's on sale at your local grocery stores, so you know where to get main ingredients on sale. Now you're ready to shop!

ESTABLISH A COOKING DAY

When you have all the necessary ingredients on hand, take one day that works for your schedule and cook a few meals in advance. They can be stored in serving containers in the fridge, or frozen to be reheated during the week. Alternatively, you can do basic prep for a few meals—chopping vegetables, slicing meat, or premixing sauces or marinades, for example—to make cooking during the week a little easier. It may seem like a lot of work to do in one day, but it will make your week easier when it comes to mealtimes. If you have kids, get them involved. If they feel like they're part of this process, they may even want to help you shop, cook and clean up!

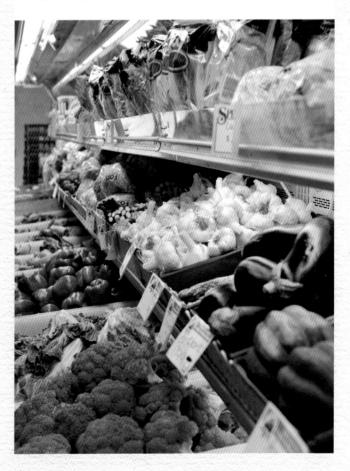

THE GROCERY LIST

I like to shop from left to right, because that's how I enter the door at my local store. I know the store so well that I can write my shopping list to follow the order I'll find things in as I go through the aisles. You can create a method that works well for you. No matter what you are preparing for the week, though, your list will include *protein*, *carbohydrates* and *fat*.

When shopping for protein—i.e., meat, fish, or eggs—try to select products that are sustainably raised, such as grass-fed beef or free-range poultry. Always choose wild-caught fish if available, whether fresh, frozen, or canned.

PROTEINS SHOULD INCLUDE:	**Bacon** (nitrate free); **Beef** (flank, chuck, sirloin, tenderloin, or other lean cuts); **Eggs; Game Meats; Fish** (fresh and canned); **Lean Veal; Lean Pork; Poultry; Rabbit; Quail**
CARBO-HYDRATES SHOULD INCLUDE:	**Dried Fruit** (unsweetened); **Fermented Foods; Fresh Fruit** (apples, apricots, berries, figs, grapefruit, kiwifruit, lemons, limes, melons, nectarines, oranges, peaches, pears, plums, pomegranates, tangerines, watermelon); **Green and Colorful Vegetables;** (asparagus, broccoli, cabbage, cauliflower, celery, collard greens, eggplant, endive, fennel, kale, lettuce, mustard greens, peppers, pumpkin, spinach, tomato); **Mushrooms; Root and Stem Vegetables** (artichokes, carrots, fennel, garlic, ginger, horseradish, onions, parsnips, sweet potatoes/yams, turnips)
FATS SHOULD INCLUDE:	**Avocados; Butter** (unsalted, or ghee—clarified butter); **Coconut Oil; Coconut flakes** (unsweetened); **Nuts and Seeds** (almonds, Brazil nuts, cashews, hazelnuts, macadamias, pecans, pine nuts, pistachios, pumpkin seeds, sunflower seeds, walnuts); **Nut Butters** (almond butter, cashew butter, sunflower butter); **Olive Oil**

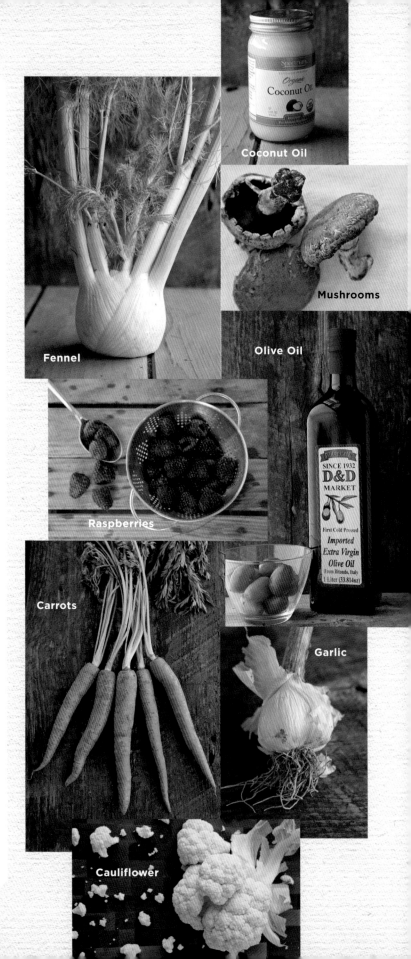

Coconut Oil

Mushrooms

Fennel

Olive Oil

Raspberries

Carrots

Garlic

Cauliflower

KEEPING YOUR ITALIAN KITCHEN PALEO

As an Italian following the Paleo lifestyle, there are pantry and refrigerated items I keep handy at all times. The following are some of my best stocking-up tips, shopping ideas and other helpful hints.

THE WELL-STOCKED PALEO ITALIAN PANTRY

Almonds Available raw, whole, sliced, chopped, smoked, in paste, blanched, and roasted and salted. Almonds are loaded with good stuff; they contain calcium, fiber, folic acid, magnesium, potassium, riboflavin and vitamin E. Toast them to intensify flavor and add satisfying crunch.

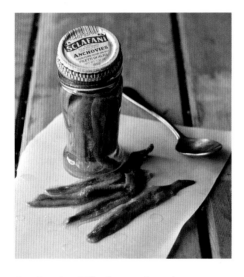

Anchovies Whether you love them or think you're not a fan, keep a container in the pantry and have a jar or tube handy in the refrigerator. Anchovies make a great pizza topping, go well on antipasti, and add depth to dressing, marinades and sauces.

Baking staples I am a pretty basic baker, but I love to make custards, biscotti and other recipes in this book. My baking staples include raw nuts, baking soda, baking powder, almond butter or other nut butter, honey, maple syrup, coconut milk, creamed coconut, arrowroot powder, palm shortening, unsweetened cocoa powder, unsweetened shredded coconut flakes, vanilla extract and other extracts, unsweetened chocolate chips, dark chocolate and canned pumpkin.

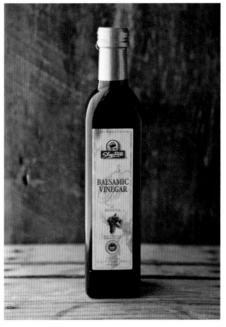

Balsamic vinegar This special type of vinegar from Modena achieves its beautiful color and depth of flavor only after spending years in wooden barrels, where becomes concentrated into a complex syrup. Drizzle balsamic vinegar over figs or strawberries (or, if you occasionally eat cheese, over Parmigiano-Reggiano) for fantastic flavor combinations.

Broth or stock Although homemade is always best, it's a good idea to keep cans or boxes of low-sodium all-natural broth handy in your pantry. If you go the homemade route, double or triple the batch and freeze the extra in containers. Broth is an essential base for soups, stews, sauces, and gravies.

Canned fish Canned tuna and salmon add a high-protein boost to salads and antipasti. They can also serve as the main ingredient in dishes like salmon cakes.

Capers Often mistaken for berries, capers are actually tiny flower buds from a bush that grows in the Mediterranean. They're typically pickled in vinegary brine or sometimes packed in salt. For something so small, they add big, pungent flavor to sauces, condiments, and meat and vegetable dishes.

Eggplant The versatile eggplant can be baked, boiled or fried. Take care when frying, though, as it can absorb a lot of oil! To minimize this, coat eggplant slices well with batter or crumbs before sliding them into hot oil.

Flours Recipes in this book call for almond flour or meal, coconut flour, tapioca flour and other nut flours in place of wheat flour for pasta, baking and cooking. Follow the instructions carefully, as these flours are not interchangeable and conversion amounts vary.

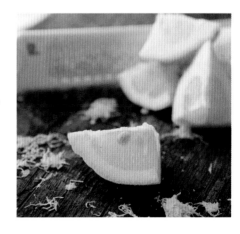

Lemons Lemons add bright flavor to a wide range of dishes, from sweet to savory. This juicy, acidic fruit is also an important ingredient in drinks, including limoncello, the famous lemon liqueur from southern Italy.

Fresh Italian herbs Fresh herbs are always preferable to dried. Use them as often as you can.

Flat-leaf parsley Also known as "Italian parsley," the flavor and aroma profile of this herb is green and vegetative. It goes particularly well in egg dishes, soups, stews, stocks and in combination with other herbs to bring out their flavor. With its vibrant green color, parsley also adds visual appeal to many dishes.

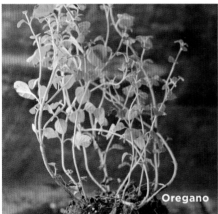
Flat-leaf Parsley

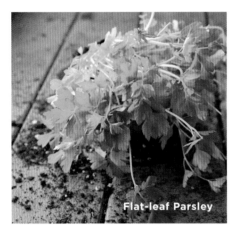
Oregano

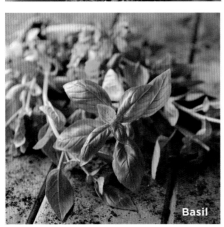
Basil

Oregano Used liberally in Italian cuisine, oregano is strongly aromatic and slightly bitter. Its pungent flavor is composed of earthy or musty, green, and minty notes.

Basil Used in tomato sauces, pestos, and Italian seasonings, basil is highly aromatic and slightly bitter, with notes of green grass, hay, and mint. Early Romans made basil a symbol of love and fertility; young Italian suitors wore sprigs of it to indicate that they were seeking marriage.

Rosemary Rosemary is popular in seasoning blends for meats and Mediterranean cuisines. It has a distinctive pine-woody aroma and a fresh, bittersweet flavor.

Sage Fragrant, with astringent savory notes, sage is ideal for flavoring pork, beef, poultry, lamb, tomatoes, squash, and much more. Traditionally, sage was prized not only as a seasoning, but for its healing properties as well.

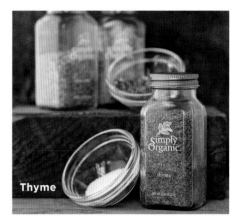
Thyme

Dried Italian herbs and seasonings Keep fresh herbs on hand when possible, but *always* stock dried herbs and seasonings. Dried basil, parsley, thyme, oregano, rosemary, sage, red pepper flakes, whole black pepper, and sea salt are the dried herbs and seasonings I use on a regular basis.

A HANDY GUIDE FOR COMMON DRIED SEASONINGS TO FOOD PAIRINGS	
Basil	Tomatoes, salads, eggs, fish, chicken, lamb, garlic
Bay Leaf	Soups, sauces
Cayenne	Wings, chicken, eggs, pizza
Celery Salt	Chicken, cabbage, hot dogs, potato salad, sautéed onions
Chives	Eggs, fish, chicken, soups, potatoes, cheeses
Cilantro	Salsa, Mexican cuisine, salads, fish, shellfish, chicken
Coriander	Meats, chicken, seafood, and Mexican, Latin, Caribbean recipes
Cumin	Chili, sausages, stews, eggs, and Mexican, Latin, Caribbean recipes
Dill	Leaves or seeds in soups, salads, potato salad, fish, shellfish, shrimp, tuna fish, vegetables; seeds only with pickles or tomatoes
Garlic	Dressings, soups, meats, rubs, pasta, sauces
Marjoram	Beef, chicken, sausages, seafood, stuffing, vegetables
Mint	Beverages, desserts, lamb, sauces, soups
Mustard Seed	Meats, pickling, relishes, sauces
Nutmeg	Beverages, Swedish meatballs, cakes, cookies, squash, sweet potatoes, holiday baking
Oregano	Italian recipes, tomatoes, chicken dishes, fish
Paprika	Chicken, deviled eggs, dips, egg salad, potato salad
Parsley	Herb mixtures, Italian recipes, garnish, pasta and ravioli, sauces, soups, stews
Rosemary	Lamb, veal, beef, poultry, game, marinade, stews
Sage	Poultry, pork, stuffing, pasta, tomatoes, fry as garnish
Tarragon	Chicken, fish, eggs, salad dressings, sauces, tomatoes
Thyme	Fish, chicken, meats, stews, soups, tomatoes

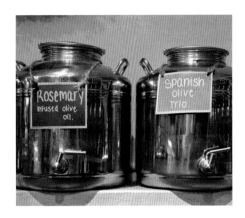

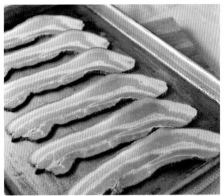

Oil Olive oil is an essential in Italian cuisine. I use regular olive oil for cooking, as it is less expensive than extra-virgin and great for high heat. Splurge on high-quality extra-virgin olive oil for dressings and for drizzling over dishes such as vegetables, antipasti, pasta, etc., and keep it close at hand. Other oil choices for cooking include coconut oil, palm oil and nut oils.

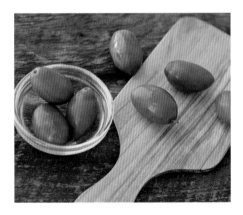

Olives Along with grapes and bread, olives were one of the three sacred elements of Roman cuisine. They remain an important ingredient in Italian food, appearing in everything from antipasti to main-course dishes.

Onions You'll know an Italian kitchen by the scent of onions and garlic cooking—two of the most important ingredients in any Italian dish. Yellow and white onions are mostly used for sauces, sautés, soups or stews and other cooking; red onions are often thinly sliced and eaten raw with salads, as they have a milder flavor and look beautiful on a large platter.

Pancetta Pancetta, which is similar to bacon, is taken from the belly of the pig. The pork is rubbed with salt and spices; it is then cured for a couple of weeks.

You may find pancetta at your local Italian market or grocery stores in one of two forms:
- Sliced thin or thick like bacon. This type of pancetta is suitable for frying like bacon, wrapping meatloaf or just eating out of the package. I often slice it into strips after cooking and add it to an Italian salad or antipasto plate.
- In rounds cut from a roll. This type is the easiest to find. It works well diced and cooked up to flavor any Italian dish, especially Amatriciana sauce.

Pine nuts Italian pine nuts have a delicate flavor and are used in sweet and savory dishes. They are probably best known as one of the principal ingredients in Italian pesto.

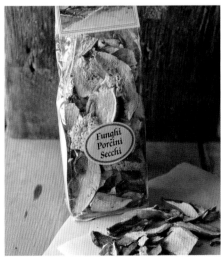

Porcini mushrooms These wild mushrooms are usually found in dried form. Their meaty texture and nutty, earthy flavor makes them particularly good in soups, risotto, stuffing and stews, and with braised meats. Before using in recipes, soak dried porcinis in hot water for about 20 minutes, and add some of the soaking water to the dish.

Prosciutto di Parma Like Parmesan cheese, this is a classic ingredient from the Emilia-Romagna region of Italy in the province of Parma. Prosciutto means "ham" in Italian, and salt-cured prosciutto di Parma is the best available. The secret is the pigs' diet of chestnuts and whey.

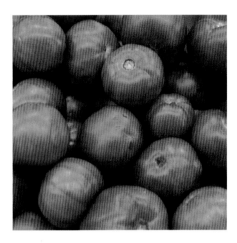

Tomatoes Delectable raw or cooked, tomatoes pair beautifully with so many foods and flavors: cheeses, meats, onions, garlic, peppers and herbs; pizza, pastas, salsas, salads, soups, stews and on and on. For a well-stocked pantry, keep whole, diced, petite diced, crushed and stewed tomatoes (as well as tomato sauce and paste) on hand for everyday cooking.

ESSENTIAL TOOLS FOR ITALIAN COOKING

When I was little, we didn't have the fancy appliances available in modern kitchens. Even now, when you travel through Italy, you'll see women making pasta and bread by hand. Gadgets are fun to use, but you don't need them to make healthy Italian Paleo recipes. That said, I think every Italian cook, whether professional or amateur, should have handy at all times a strainer, a pizza stone, a mandoline, an espresso maker, a large pot on the stove and a glass of wine!

The following are tools and appliances that I consider essential. I keep them close at hand and use them often. The items are listed in order of importance, by my estimation. Other tools, such as a spiral vegetable slicer, food mill, handheld immersion blender or a pastry cutter, are nice to have, but I don't include them in my "necessary" list. Italian cooks have done without them for centuries, and there are other ways to get the job done.

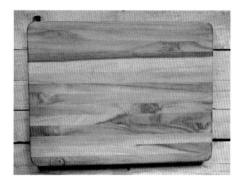

Large wood block and poultry-safe cutting boards You only need one large wooden board for chopping vegetables, but keep several polypropylene boards handy for cutting poultry and other meats.

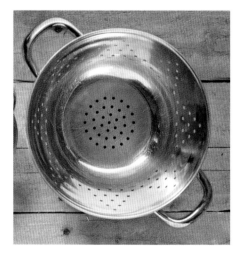

Colander This is an essential kitchen tool. You can use it for draining vegetables and fruits after washing, draining boiled foods, or as an attractive way to store fruits like apples.

A four- or six-quart / liter saucepan to keep on your stove at all times This size pot is perfect for cooking meatballs or braising chicken or short ribs. Keep it handy.

An eight- to twelve-quart / liter pot for soups, sauces and stews An Italian cook keeps a pot of sauce, a soup or a stew going on the stove at all times.

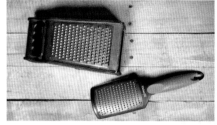

Grater/zester (either a box grater or the grater disk of a food processor) I find I use my grater frequently for grating garlic, ginger, lemons and Parmesan cheese, and for the dark chocolate on my favorite desserts.

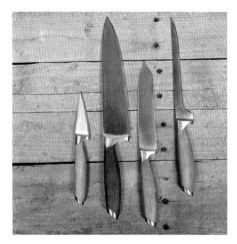

A good set of knives, including a chef's knife and paring knife See page 22.

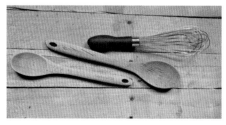

Wooden spoons, ladles, kitchen scissors, whisk, can opener I keep these utensils on my counter for easy access.

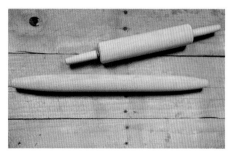

Wooden rolling pin When I was a little girl, using the rolling pin was my biggest thrill. I loved rolling out the dough for pies with my Nana. I still have the one we used together fifty years ago!

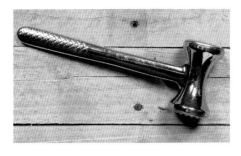

Meat tenderizer or mallet Sure, you can use a cup, a wine bottle, a hammer or some other household item to tenderize your meat—but why not get a mallet? They're not very expensive, and they make short and easy work of thinning out a flank steak or chicken breast.

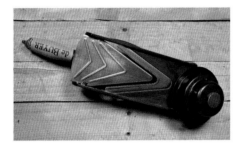

Mandoline I love my mandoline. I use it to slice sweet potatoes and other vegetables. Of course, a chef's knife works too, but a mandoline makes perfect, consistently sized slices every time.

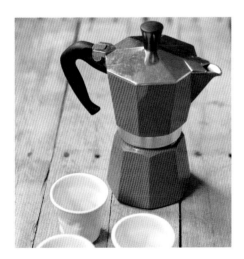

Espresso maker You don't need a fancy espresso maker that takes up your entire counter. All you need is a stove-top espresso maker like the Moka Express from Bialetti. These come in different colors and sizes, and are very affordable.

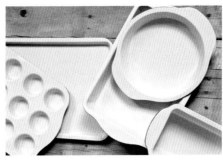

Baking pans Find a nice starter kit that includes a variety of baking pans.

Timer Even if your stove has a timer, it's wise to keep a portable one handy if you like to multi-task while you cook. Setting a timer on your phone works well, too!

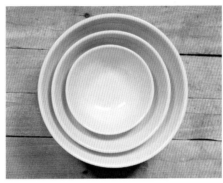

Mixing bowls Find a set of nesting mixing bowls of glass, plastic, metal, or ceramic. They're easy to stack and keep at arm's reach, and they come in very handy from breakfast to dinner and dessert!

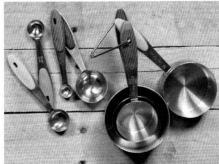

Measuring cups and spoons Nana never used measuring cups or spoons when cooking, but she always used them for baking. You should have a set of cups going from ⅛ cup to 1 cup, and a set of spoons from ⅛ tsp to 1 Tbsp.

ADDITIONAL TOOLS, POTS, PANS, BAKING DISHES, AND UTENSILS

The following is a list of all the items that I use in my kitchen. While they're nice to have, they're not strictly necessary for Italian cooking, or even for cooking in general. Keep an eye out for these items at tag sales and consignment shops rather than going out of your way to buy them new.

- Baking dishes
- Baking sheets
- Blender
- Cast-iron skillet
- Food processor
- Hand mixer
- Immersion blender
- Knife sharpener
- Muffin tins
- Rubber spatulas
- Stand mixer
- Large stockpot
- Saucepans of different sizes
- Oven-safe skillet (sauté pan)
- Tongs
- Meat thermometer

A WORD ABOUT KNIVES

A good knife is essential for cooking, and using the correct knife for the task makes everything easier. Always keep your knives clean and sharp. I use Schmidt knives; the following describes my favorites and their uses.

Chef's knife If you have to choose only one knife, get an 8- or 10-inch (20- to 25-cm) chef's knife. It's the most universal knife in the kitchen, designed for all cutting tasks. Because the blade is curved, you can rock it back and forth on the cutting board as you chop herbs or vegetables. The weight of the blade allows you to cut meat off the bone as if you were using a cleaver. Ideal for: cutting raw meat, any meat with bones, racks, large fruits, large vegetables and other large items.

Paring knife or bird's-beak paring knife A paring knife is a small knife with a 2- or 3-inch (5- to 8-cm) blade. The curved blade of a bird's-beak knife makes it well suited for delicate cutting. Ideal for: peeling pears and potatoes, deseeding peppers, deveining shrimp, or making radish roses.

Utility knife Like a chef's knife, your utility knife is always there with you in the trenches. Midway in size between a chef's knife and a paring knife, it can get a lot of jobs done. Ideal for: larger and firmer vegetables broccoli or carrots, larger fruits like melons, sandwich meats.

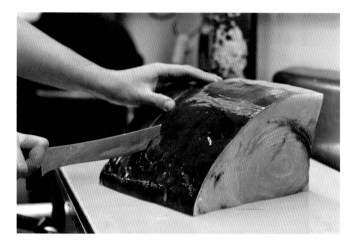

Slicer or carver You don't need a hunk of a blade to cut through a hunk of meat. For a roast, a rack or a bird, use a slicer or carving knife—the cutlery of carnivores. Long, with a blade that's either serrated or straight, a carver is the knife you need for tearing through a turkey and slicing meat as thin as you need. Ideal for: turkey, roast beef, ham, and anything else meaty and yummy.

Santoku The santoku is the Japanese version of a chef's knife. It's typically straighter and lighter than a Western-style chef's knife, but just as versatile. Ideal for: vegetables, fish, boneless chicken and thin-boned meats.

Petite chef's knife A petite chef's knife has the same shape and heft as a traditional chef's knife, but with a smaller blade—about 6 in (15 cm)—so it's better suited for smaller jobs. Ideal for: cutting raw meat, any meat with bones, fruits and vegetables.

Tomato knife Put too much pressure on a tomato and you'll get tomato sauce! A tomato knife has fine serrations that can pierce the skin and cut through the fruit without crushing it or creating soft spots. Ideal for: tomatoes and other soft fruits and vegetables.

Boning knife Dealing with bones is no fun, but the right knife makes removing them a lot easier. Boning knives are tough, but thin and flexible enough to get into small spaces. Stiffer boning knives work well for beef and pork, whereas a more flexible blade is better for boning fish and poultry. Ideal for: removing bones from meat, poultry, and fish.

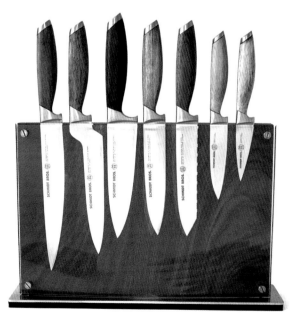

Adapted with permission from Schmidt Brothers Cutlery.

COOKING METHODS & TIPS

Always select the correct cooking method, as your choice will determine the texture, appearance and flavor of the foods you prepare. Understanding the basic cooking methods will help ensure your success in the kitchen.

Braising A slow, moist-heat cooking method in which foods are cooked in liquid in a tightly covered pot or dish for a long period of time. Braising is a good way to prepare a tough cut of meat or bone-in chicken.

Broiling A high-heat cooking method that sears the surface of the food. Usually done in the oven using the broiler setting. Always stay near your oven when broiling, and keep the door slightly ajar.

Grilling Cooking food over charcoal, wood or gas flames. Food can be grilled indoors on a grill pan or outdoors on a full grill.

Frying Cooking food in a skillet or pan over direct heat, usually in hot oil.

Roasting A dry heat cooking method in which heat is not transferred through a liquid medium as when braising or stewing. Roasting develops complex flavors and aromas.

Stewing A slow moist-heat cooking method using a pot with a lid. Ingredients are simmered until they are soft and the flavors have mingled thoroughly.

Stir-frying A quick dry-heat cooking method using a lightly oiled pan. Stir-frying uses high heat while continuously tossing ingredients.

Sautéing A high-heat method using fat such as butter or oil. I use the combination of butter and oil to achieve a crust on meat or poultry. No liquid is used with this method.

MEAT COOKING TEMPERATURES

I often refer to these guidelines when cooking meats. Remember to always let the meat rest for a few minutes before slicing or serving; the meat will continue to cook as it sits.

BEEF, LAMB OR PORK ROASTS, STEAKS AND CHOPS

Rare	120–125°F (50–52°C)
Medium-rare	130–135°F (55–57°C)
Medium	140–145°F (60–63°C)
Medium-well	150–155°F (65°–70°C)
Well done	160°F (72°C) and above

Ground Meat	160–165°F (72–75°C)
Poultry and Turkey	165°F (75°C)
Pork Ribs, Shoulders & Beef Brisket	160°F (72°C) and above
Sausage (raw)	160°F (72°C)
Ham (raw)	160°F (72°C)
Ham (pre-cooked)	140°F (60°C)
Fish (steaks, fillet or whole)	140°F (60°C)
Tuna, Marlin & Swordfish	125°F (52°C)

QUANTITY EQUIVALENTS

3 teaspoons	1 tablespoon
2 tablespoons	⅛ cup
5 tablespoons plus 1 teaspoon	⅓ cup
8 tablespoons	½ cup
12 tablespoons	¾ cup
16 tablespoons	1 cup

1 ounce	2 tablespoons of fat or liquid
4 ounces	½ cup
8 ounces	1 cup
16 ounces	2 cups, or one pint
2 cups liquid	1 pound
2 pints	1 quart
1 quart	4 cups

A pinch of salt = the amount of salt that you can fit between your finger and thumb	
A speck = less than ⅛ teaspoon	

METRIC CONVERSIONS

Volume (for fluid measurements only; dry ingredients are measured by weight):	
1 teaspoon	5 grams
1 tablespoon	15 grams
⅛ cup (1 ounce)	30 ml
¼ cup (2 ounces)	65 ml
⅓ cup (2.6 ounces)	80 ml
½ cup (4 ounces)	125 ml
¾ cup (6 ounces)	185 ml
1 cup (8 ounces)	250 ml
2 cups (1 pint)	500 ml
4 cups (1 quart)	1 liter
8 cups (1 gallon)	3.7 liters

Weight:	
1 ounce	50 grams
4 ounces (¼ pound)	100 grams
8 ounces (½ pound)	250 grams
16 ounces (1 pound)	500 grams

MINCING ONIONS

MINCING GARLIC

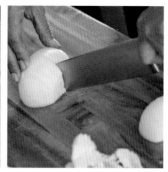

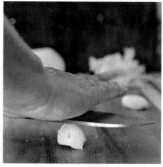

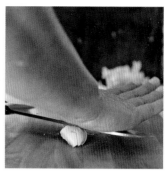

Cut a peeled onion through the middle, top to bottom.

Cut the half into vertical slices.

Carefully place a clove under the flat side of a kitchen knife blade.

Press down on the flat of the blade with the palm of your hand to split the skin of the clove.

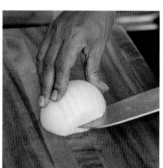

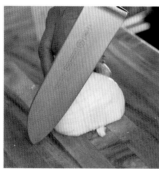

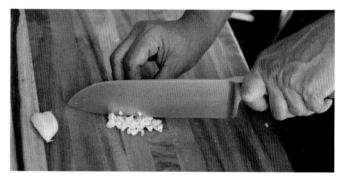

Holding the slices together, carefully cut the onion into horizontal slices.

Cut the onion into vertical slices again, this time at 90 degrees to the original vertical slices.

Remove the skin and mince the garlic into small pieces.

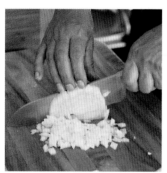

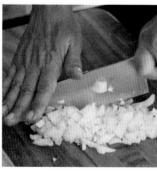

The mincing in progress.

Cut the roughly chopped pieces into as fine a mince as desired.

CINDY'S TOP TWENTY COOKING TIPS

Here are some tips to help you make everyday cooking and entertaining easy and stress-free! A little advance planning and cleaning up as you cook will go a long way toward success in the kitchen.

1 Complete basic dinner preparations the night before or in the morning to make cooking the meal less stressful.

2 Making sauce or stock? Prepare in large quantities and freeze in quart containers or freezer-safe bags.

3 Avoid the temptation to test new recipes when entertaining. Stick to the recipes you can execute without a hitch, and save experiments for casual meals.

4 Cook spaghetti squash to *al dente* in advance. Just before serving time, toss in a large skillet with a little oil, salt and pepper to warm through and finish cooking.

5 Bring eggs and butter to room temperature before using them for baking.

6 Allow meat to rest after grilling or roasting. This will allow the juices to redistribute and keep the meat moist.

7 Never overcrowd the pan when sautéing—you'll end up with steamed food. Work in batches if needed, and keep a warm plate in the oven to keep sautéed items hot.

8 When you go shopping, always take a list, and never go hungry.

9 Always make sure your knives are sharp.

10 For best results, use exact

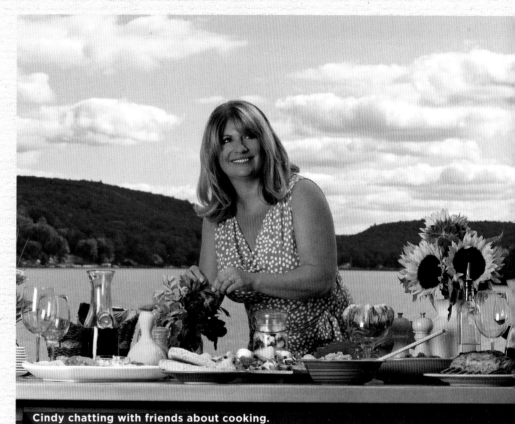

Cindy chatting with friends about cooking.

measurements when baking.

11 To get the most juice from a lemon or lime, roll it on the counter under your palm before squeezing.

12 Clean as you cook!

13 Cook with your favorite music playing and a glass of wine in hand. Enjoy your time in the kitchen.

14 To prevent an egg from cracking while boiling, start with cold water and add in a capful of distilled vinegar.

15 Iceberg lettuce will stay fresh in the refrigerator if you wrap it in a clean, dry paper towel and store it in a sealed plastic bag.

16 Always heat the pan, then add oil.

17 A great way to test whether your oil is hot enough is to place the end of a wooden spoon in the pan. If you see bubbles form around the wood, you're ready to go.

18 Use sea salt or kosher salt, which have more flavor and mineral benefits, rather than iodized salt.

19 Always have fresh salami, prosciutto, mortadella, olives, anchovies and nuts handy to make a quick antipasto to serve guests.

20 Read the entire recipe before you start to cook!

BASIC RECIPES

Spending a little time preparing ingredients that you will use often and storing them is part of keeping your ingredients as fresh and pure as possible. Homemade foods also make great gifts. I just love having homemade marinated vegetables on hand to serve as an appetizer, to add to my antipasto, or put on top of a salad.

Likewise, homemade stock or broth adds a depth of flavor to soups and stews that you just can't get out of a can or carton. Most Italians make stock and broth from scratch using meaty bones. Your butcher may sell soup bones; you can also just tell them that you're making stock and ask them for any bones they may have on hand. Just remember not to oversalt your stock! It's better to add seasoning to soups, stews, gravy and other dishes as they are being prepared.

ITALIAN PICKLED VEGETABLES

My grandfather had a large vegetable garden. When the vegetables were ready, Nana and I would make a bunch of jars of pickled vegetables to be served on an antipasto platter at Sunday dinner. Nana insisted that all of the vegetables, except for the cauliflower and artichokes, had to be the same shape. Really, though, you can cut them any way you want. I like to slice some and cut others into matchsticks.

PREP TIME: 30 MINUTES
COOK TIME: 3 MINUTES
MAKES: 4 CUPS

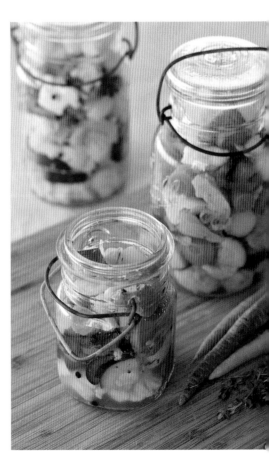

1 cup (100 g) cauliflower, broken into small florets
2 medium carrots, peeled and sliced
1 cup (100 g) button or pearl onions
1 red bell pepper, sliced or cut into chunks
2 medium zucchini, sliced
1 cup (150 g) marinated artichoke hearts, quartered
2 cloves garlic, chopped
½ cup (125 ml) extra-virgin olive oil
1 cup (250 ml) white wine vinegar
¼ cup (65 ml) fresh lemon juice
1 tablespoon dried oregano
½ teaspoon dried rosemary
½ teaspoon dried thyme
2 teaspoons sea salt
2 teaspoons whole black peppercorns
Dried red pepper flakes (optional)

Bring a large pot of water to a boil. Add the cauliflower, carrots, onions, pepper and zucchini and blanch for 3 minutes. Remove from pot and drain, then place in a large bowl. The vegetables should still be crisp.

Add the artichokes.

In a separate bowl, combine the garlic, extra-virgin olive oil, white wine vinegar, lemon juice, oregano, rosemary, thyme, salt and pepper, then whisk together.

Pour over vegetables and, using a wooden spoon, stir to combine. Cover and refrigerate overnight.

Ladle the pickles into clean jars. Add a pinch of red pepper flakes, if using, to each jar, then cover tightly with a lid.

These pickles will last for 1 week in the refrigerator.

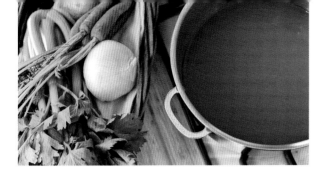

CHICKEN BROTH

Buying canned chicken broth is easy, sure—but when you make your own, you know exactly what went into it. Homemade chicken broth does take a little planning and time, but you can make several quarts and freeze them for later use. All you need to do is defrost them before adding your homemade broth to soups, sauces, gravy and other recipes.

PREP TIME: 15 MINUTES
COOK TIME: 3½ HOURS
MAKES: 6 CUPS

2 large roasting chickens (about 4–5 lbs / 2 kg total)
2 large yellow onions, left unpeeled and quartered
3 carrots, left unpeeled and halved
3 stalks celery with leaves, cut into thirds
1 leek, white part only, cut in half lengthwise
2 or 3 bay leaves
10 sprigs fresh thyme
1 cup (30 g) fresh parsley (both stems and leaves)
2 large cloves garlic, peeled
2 tablespoons sea salt
1 tablespoon whole black peppercorns
1 gallon (3.75 liters) water

Place all ingredients in a stockpot, large soup pot or Dutch oven. Bring to a boil, then reduce heat to medium-low.

Use a large spoon or fine-mesh strainer to skim the scum from the surface of the broth. Cover and allow to simmer for 3 hours, skimming every 30 minutes. Remove broth from heat.

Place a sieve over a large bowl and pour the stock through, reserving the broth in the bowl and discarding all solids. Chill the broth overnight in one or more containers. The next day, remove the fat that has risen to the surface. The broth may be used immediately or frozen for later use.

VEAL STOCK

The extra flavor of veal stock enhances osso buco and adds depth to any braised dish. You can substitute other meat bones and follow the same recipe; either way will make a richly flavored stock that brings out the best in any recipe.

PREP TIME: 15 MINUTES
COOK TIME: 6 TO 12 HOURS
MAKES: 5 CUPS

5 lbs (2.25 kg) meaty veal bones and veal knuckles, cut into pieces
2 to 3 tablespoons olive oil or melted coconut oil
1 tablespoon unsalted butter
2 tablespoons tomato paste
2 large yellow onions, chopped
3 large carrots, chopped
3 celery ribs, chopped
2 bay leaves
5 cloves garlic, peeled
½ cup (125 ml) red wine
1 gallon (3.75 liters) cold water
5 fresh thyme sprigs
1 cup (30 g) fresh flat-leaf parsley, stems and leaves
1 tablespoon whole black peppercorns

Preheat oven to 425°F (220°C).
Line a baking sheet with foil, then brush with oil to coat.
Place veal bones or knuckles on the pan in a single layer. Bake for 45 minutes, turning once halfway through.
Place a large stockpot or Dutch oven over medium heat. Melt the butter, then add the tomato paste, spreading it around the pan with a wooden spoon.
Next add the onions, carrots, celery, bay leaves and garlic. Cook together for about 5 minutes, then stir in the red wine.
Add the bones to the pot, then the water, thyme, parsley and whole peppercorns.
Cover, lower the heat to medium-low and bring to a simmer. When it just begins to boil, reduce the heat to low. Skim off any foam that has risen to the top of the pot.
Cover and simmer for at least 6 hours—and preferably longer; up to 12 hours—skimming every 45 minutes. Remove from heat.
Line a strainer with cheesecloth and place over a large bowl. Pour the contents of the pot through the strainer, reserving the stock and discarding the bones and other solids.
Cover the bowl and refrigerate until completely cooled. Discard any fat that congeals on top of the liquid. The stock can be used immediately or frozen for future use.

CINDY'S TIP
If you use a pressure cooker, this stock only takes 2 hours to cook.

SAUCES & CONDIMENTS

One sign of an authentic Italian kitchen is the large pot of sauce that will be simmering on the stove. I love making triple batches of sauce so I have extra to divide up and freeze for later use or to give away. These sauces will make your house smell glorious as they cook. Let the sauce simmer all day to make it truly unforgettable.

Here's a tip for adding extra flavor to any tomato sauce: heat some olive oil in the pot you plan to use for cooking the sauce. Add 2 tablespoons of chopped pancetta and 2 tablespoons of diced onions. Sauté until the pancetta gets crispy, then remove the onion and pancetta with a slotted spoon and drain on a paper-towel-lined plate. Leave the flavored oil in the pot and start cooking your sauce—it will be even better than usual. Topping your final dish with the crispy pancetta and onion will add a little extra Italian flair.

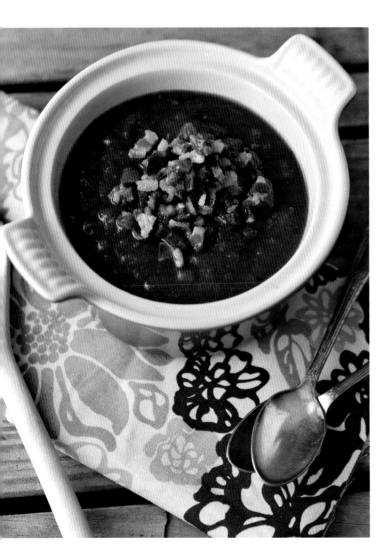

AMATRICIANA SAUCE

This popular sauce can be found in many Roman restaurants. Amatriciana is traditionally made with pork jowl, but I like to use pancetta or other non-smoked bacon. This sauce goes great with braised short ribs.

PREP TIME: 15 MINUTES
COOK TIME: 30 MINUTES
** TO 1 HOUR**
MAKES: 3 CUPS (750 ML)

2 tablespoons olive oil
5 slices pancetta or uncured
  bacon, diced
1 small yellow onion,
  chopped
2 cloves garlic, minced
½ teaspoon dried red pep-
  per flakes
1 teaspoon sea salt
¾ teaspoon freshly ground
  black pepper
One 28-oz (800-g) can
  crushed tomatoes
1 teaspoon dried basil

Heat the olive oil in a large pot over medium heat. Add pancetta or bacon and sauté until crisp and golden, about 5 to 7 minutes.

Stir in the onion, garlic and red pepper flakes. Cook for about 5 minutes more.

Add the salt, pepper, crushed tomatoes and basil, and stir to combine.

Bring the sauce to a boil, then immediately reduce heat to low. Cover and simmer for 15 to 20 minutes, stirring occasionally, until the sauce thickens.

CINDY'S TIP
For greater depth of flavor, add a splash of the red wine that you will be enjoying with dinner.

BASIC MARINARA SAUCE

I normally double or triple this recipe and freeze portions in individual containers. I try to make it basic; depending on the recipe I add it to, I can add more flavors such as wine or chicken broth. When making marinara, remember that dried herbs hold their flavor and color through slow cooking, but fresh herbs should not be added until the end of the cooking process. Stir them in just before serving. If you have fresh tomatoes rather than canned, use 3 pounds (1.4 kg) for a single recipe.

CINDY'S TIP
To incorporate the tomato paste into the sauce smoothly, press it against the side of the pan with the back of a spoon before stirring it in.

PREP TIME: 15 MINUTES
COOK TIME: 35 MINUTES
MAKES: 3½ CUPS (900 ML)

⅓ cup (80 ml) olive oil
½ cup (75 g) finely diced yellow onion
2 cloves garlic, minced
¼ teaspoon dried red pepper flakes
4 cups (1 liter) canned San Marzano
   Italian plum tomatoes in juice or
   crushed tomatoes
One 6-oz (175-g) can tomato paste
1½ teaspoon sea salt
1 teaspoon freshly ground black pepper
2 teaspoons dried basil
1 teaspoon dried oregano
1 teaspoon dried parsley
½ teaspoon dried thyme

Place a large pot over medium-high heat. When hot, add the olive oil, then add the onion and cook for 30 seconds. Reduce heat to medium and add the garlic and red pepper flakes.

Add the tomatoes and bring to a boil, then add the tomato paste a teaspoonful at a time. Fill the tomato paste can with hot water and stir with the teaspoon (to loosen all of the paste), then pour into the pot.

Add the salt and seasonings then stir using a wooden spoon.

Bring to a boil, then cover and reduce to a simmer. Let cook for 15 to 30 minutes. Check seasoning, adding more herbs or salt as needed.

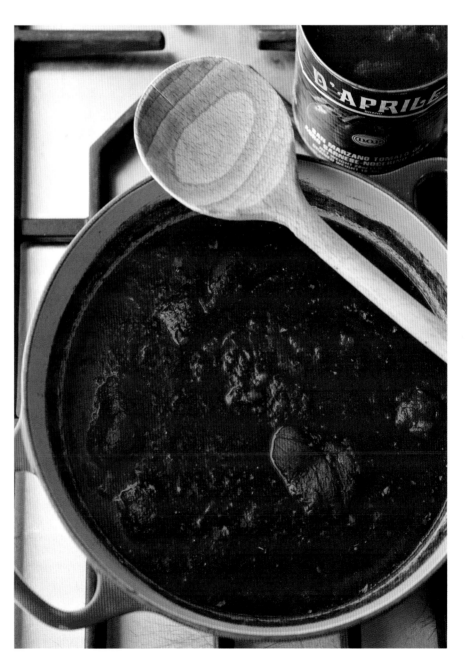

TUSCAN-STYLE BOLOGNESE

I love the satisfying texture of this Bolognese. In Italy, where it is called *sugo di carne* (simple meat sauce), it contains a lot of meat and just a little sauce. Tuscan-style Bolognese can be found throughout Tuscany and central Italy.

PREP TIME: 20 MINUTES
COOK TIME: 1½ HOURS
MAKES: 4 CUPS (1 LITER)

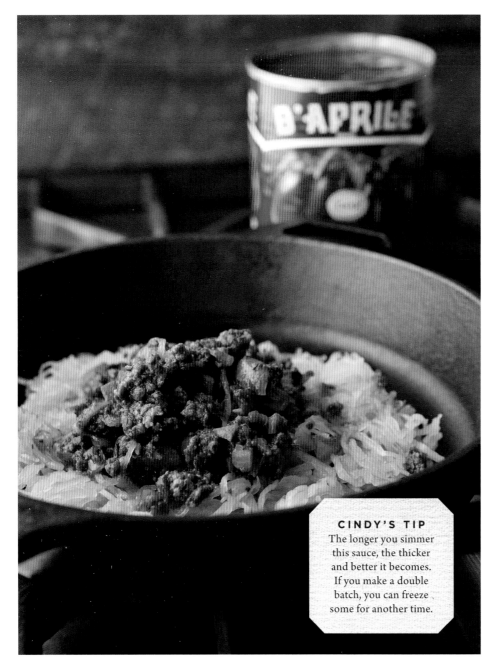

CINDY'S TIP
The longer you simmer this sauce, the thicker and better it becomes. If you make a double batch, you can freeze some for another time.

3 tablespoons unsalted butter
3 tablespoons olive oil
4 slices pancetta, chopped
1 onion, diced
1 carrot, diced
3 to 4 cloves garlic, minced
1 lb (500 g) ground beef
½ lb (225 g) ground pork
½ lb (225 g) ground veal
1 cup (250 ml) dry white wine
One 28-oz (800-g) can crushed
   tomatoes
One 6-oz (175-g) can tomato paste
1 teaspoon sea salt
¾ teaspoon freshly ground black
   pepper
1 tablespoon dried oregano
½ teaspoon dried sage
¼ teaspoon dried red pepper flakes

Place a Dutch oven or large pot over medium heat. When hot, add the butter and olive oil. Once the butter has melted, add the pancetta and cook until crisp. Use a slotted spoon to transfer to a plate lined with a paper towel.

Add the onion and carrot to the hot pan and sauté for 3 minutes. Add the garlic, beef, pork and veal. Cook for about 10 minutes, stirring often with a wooden spoon so that the meat breaks up into small pieces.

Stir in the white wine and crushed tomatoes, then bring the sauce to a boil. Mix in the tomato paste, then add the salt, pepper, oregano, sage and red pepper flakes. Stir until all of the herbs are incorporated, then add in pancetta and stir again. Lower the heat and cover. Allow sauce to simmer for at least 30 minutes, or longer if desired.

PORTOBELLO RAGÙ

I like to serve this hearty, flavorful sauce over spaghetti squash or with sautéed chicken. Though this recipe calls for dried herbs, fresh herbs can also be used; add them toward the end of the cooking process. Taste often to correct seasoning as needed.

PREP TIME: 15 MINUTES
COOK TIME: 1 HOUR
MAKES: 4 CUPS (1 LITER)

4 portobello mushrooms
¼ cup (60 ml) olive oil, divided
4 slices pancetta, chopped
1 yellow onion, diced
1½ teaspoons sea salt
1 teaspoon freshly ground black pepper
3 cloves garlic, minced
¾ cup (185 ml) dry red wine
1 teaspoon dried thyme
1 teaspoon dried sage
1 teaspoon dried rosemary
1½ teaspoons dried oregano
One 32-oz (900-g) can chopped or
    crushed tomatoes
One 6-oz (175-g) can tomato paste

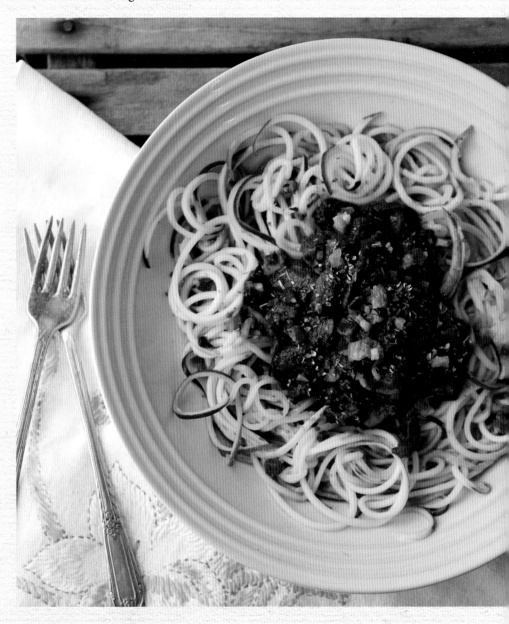

Remove the stems from the portobello mushrooms and gently scrape off the gills with a teaspoon. Coarsely chop the mushrooms. Set aside.

Place a large skillet over medium heat. Once hot, add 2 tablespoons of the olive oil, then add the pancetta and onion. Sauté, stirring often with a wooden spoon, until the pancetta is crispy. Remove the onions and pancetta using a slotted spoon and place on a plate lined with a paper towel.

Add the remaining 2 tablespoons of olive oil to the same skillet over medium-high heat. When hot, add the mushrooms and stir with a wooden spoon so that they are coated in oil. Add the salt, pepper and garlic and sauté for about 5 minutes, stirring often. Pour in the wine to deglaze the pan, scraping up the bits at the bottom of the pan and incorporating them into the wine liquid.

Stir in the thyme, sage, rosemary, oregano and tomatoes. Bring the sauce to a boil.

Add the tomato paste a spoonful at a time, pressing it against the side of the pan with the back of the spoon so that it is smoothly incorporated.

Fill the tomato paste can halfway with warm water. Stir to pick up any paste remaining in the can, then pour into the sauce. Add the cooked pancetta and onions, stir to combine, and cover. Reduce heat to low and simmer for 15 to 20 minutes, or until cooked to taste.

PALEO MAYONNAISE

Making mayonnaise with a food processor, blender or immersion blender is far easier than doing it by hand. This three-step Paleo Mayonnaise is simple and delicious. Paleo Mayonnaise goes especially well with Tuscan Turkey Burgers, Grilled Artichokes with Lemon Basil Pesto Aioli, Italian Hero Sandwiches and Venetian Potatoes. It should be kept refrigerated in a sealed container and used within 5 days.

PREP TIME: 5 MINUTES
MAKES: 1 CUP

2 egg yolks
Juice of 1 lemon (about 1 tablespoon)
½ teaspoon dried mustard
1 cup (250 ml) avocado oil
Salt and pepper, to taste

Place egg yolks, lemon juice and mustard in a food processor or blender. Blend for 30 seconds.

With the blender or food processor at low speed, slowly drizzle in the oil to create an emulsion.

Add salt and pepper to taste.

A FEW THINGS TO REMEMBER FOR A SUCCESSFUL MAYONNAISE

- Start with eggs at room temperature. I follow this rule when all other ingredients are at room temperature.
- Add oil very slowly—a teaspoonful at a time at first. If you add the oil too quickly, the mayonnaise will not thicken properly.
- Before seasoning with salt and pepper, taste the mayonnaise, then add small amounts (less than ⅛ of a teaspoon to start).

VARIATIONS TO MAKE YOUR MAYONNAISE SPECIAL

Here are some ideas for giving your mayonnaise a different taste:
- Add chopped fresh herbs or dried herbs—try dill if you're making chicken or tuna salad.
- Add a bit of hot sauce for an extra kick.
- For a Southwestern flavor, add chili powder, garlic powder and diced cilantro.
- Grated horseradish adds a nice zing.
- Add curry powder and lime juice for an East Indian taste.
- For smoky mayo, add smoked paprika and lemon juice.

CINDY'S TIP
Since I'm an avocado lover, I suggest using avocado oil in this recipe. However, olive oil adds a unique flavor and complements the mayonnaise nicely. Macadamia nut oil, a blend of coconut and olive oil, or any other healthy oil will work well too.

SALSA VERDE (GREEN SAUCE)

The bold flavor of Salsa Verde will make any dish stand out. My favorite way to serve it is with grilled flank steak, but it also goes well with chicken or seafood. Salsa Verde can be prepared the day before serving and kept refrigerated in a covered container. There are two ways to prepare Salsa Verde—one requires cooking, the other does not.

PREP TIME: 10 MINUTES
COOK TIME (FOR METHOD TWO): 6 MINUTES
MAKES: 2 CUPS (500 ML)

6 medium tomatillos, husks removed, rinsed
1 jalapeño pepper, seeded and chopped
Olive oil (for Method Two)
¼ cup (5 g) fresh cilantro, chopped
1 small onion, chopped
½ teaspoon sea salt
3 tablespoons water (for Method One)

METHOD ONE (NO-COOK VERSION)
Cut the tomatillos into quarters.

Place all ingredients in a food processor and pulse to make a chunky salsa. Taste and adjust seasonings as needed.

Transfer to a serving bowl or storage container.

METHOD TWO (BROILED VERSION)
Place the whole tomatillos and chopped jalapeño on a baking sheet and drizzle with a little olive oil.

Place in the oven under the broiler. Keeping the door slightly ajar, broil for 5 to 6 minutes, until the tomatillos begin to blister. Place all ingredients in a food processor and process until chunky.

Taste and adjust seasonings as needed.

Transfer to a serving bowl or storage container.

CINDY'S NOTE ABOUT TOMATILLOS
You might have noticed tomatillos at the market, and wondered what to do with them. These small tomato-like fruits, which are covered in a papery husk, have a lemony flavor that adds tang to any recipe. They're a wonderful addition to salsas or stews. I also like to simmer them in a slow-cooker with chicken. Tomatillos are harvested in late summer; they may be harder to find at other times of the year.

FRESH HERB BUTTER

This delectable butter adds a special Italian touch to your meal. Though it involves a bit of extra work, the smiles you'll see on the faces around your table will make it worth the effort.

PREP TIME: 10 MINUTES
MAKES: ½ CUP (125 G)

½ cup (1 stick/125 g) unsalted organic butter, at room temperature

1 tablespoon fresh basil, finely chopped

1 tablespoon fresh thyme, finely chopped

1 tablespoon fresh tarragon leaves, finely chopped

1 tablespoon fresh chives, finely chopped

Zest of 1 lemon

1 teaspoon freshly squeezed lemon juice

1 teaspoon sea salt

¼ teaspoon freshly ground black pepper

Parchment paper or waxed paper (optional)

Place the butter in a medium-sized bowl, then add the remaining ingredients.
   Mix well, at first with a fork and then with a rubber spatula.
   Transfer to a small serving bowl and cover; or place on a piece of parchment or waxed paper, roll into a cylinder and seal the ends.
   Refrigerate for 2 hours or until firm.
   Serve with grilled steak or vegetables.

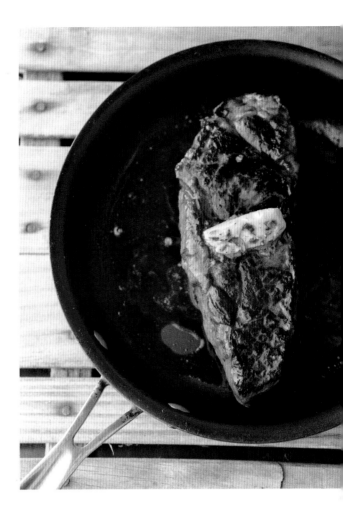

SIMPLE ITALIAN SALAD DRESSING

This wonderful Italian dressing only requires a few simple ingredients. Add your favorite Italian herbs for a personal twist!

PREP TIME: 10 MINUTES
MAKES: 1 CUP (250 ML)

1 tablespoon diced shallots

1 clove garlic, minced

Salt, to taste

Freshly ground black pepper, to taste

¼ cup (65 ml) vinegar

1 cup (250 ml) extra-virgin olive oil

Combine all ingredients in a medium-sized bowl and whisk well to blend.
   Drizzle over fresh salad greens.

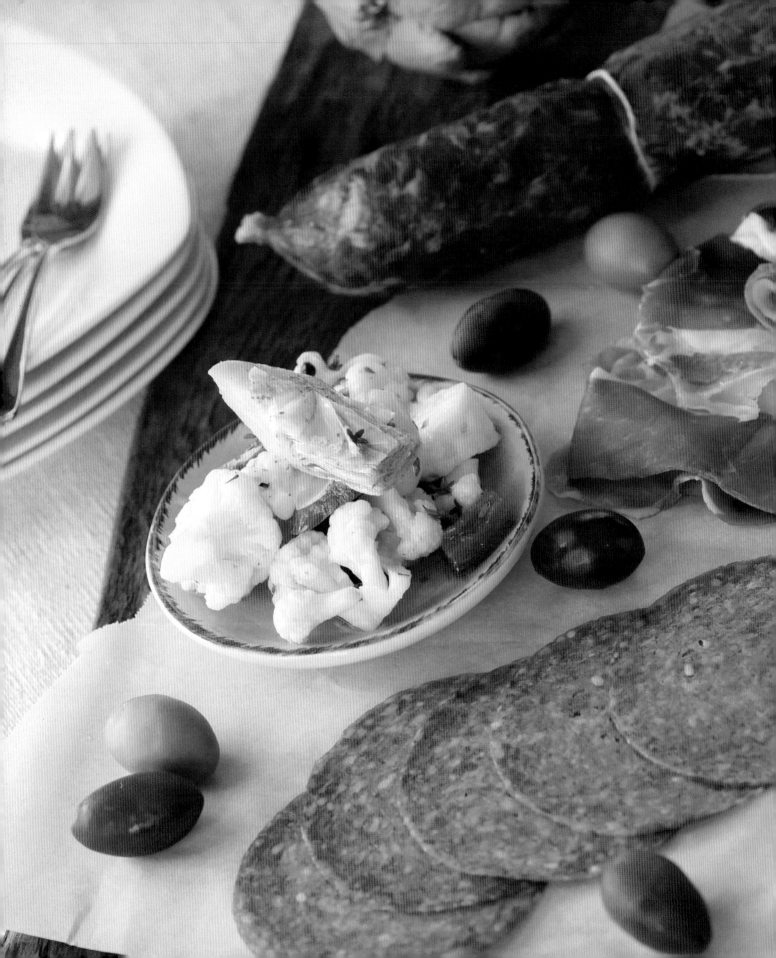

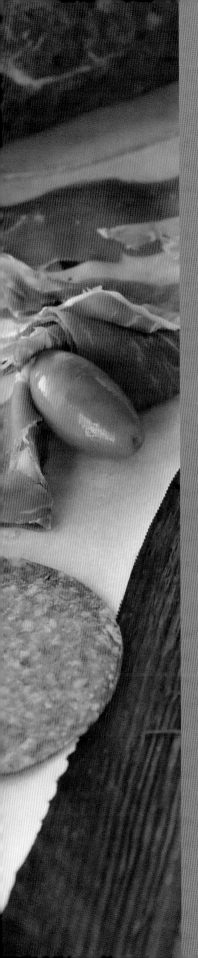

APPETIZERS
& SALADS

In an Italian household, the food starts coming out as soon
as a visiting family member or guest has been greeted.
My grandmother did it this way; my mother does it;
my sisters and I do it—it's just an Italian thing!
You'll always find fresh meats, olives, mushrooms and
vegetables in a properly stocked Italian pantry and
refrigerator. With these ingredients, making an antipasti
platter is always easy. It's a beautiful appetizer, and you can
add different ingredients to vary the colors and flavors.
The other Paleo Italian appetizers in this chapter are
great for entertaining, or for a weekend dinner or
date night. They can all be made in advance with
a few quick finishing touches. They're all favorites in
Tuscany, as well as in the homes of Italian expats.
My favorite salads are simple, yet full of flavor. Nana used
to say that salads were her way to use up leftovers over a
bowl of greens. She really had it right! You can use cooked
vegetables, leftover meats or seafood, eggs and just about
anything else to create a wonderful salad. Sometimes, if we
get last-minute company, I use this technique to be sure
there's enough food. Every Italian cook's biggest fear is the
same—running out of food! That's why we make enough
to feed an army when there are only six at the table.
The truth is we want you to take some home.

ANTIPASTO PLATTER

Literally translated, antipasti are the foods offered before a meal. The colorful antipasto platter includes a variety of meats, olives, artichokes, eggs, anchovies and other ingredients, making a veritable mini-feast. Serving an antipasto platter is a great way to get everyone socializing together.

Italians base their antipasto selections on color, flavor, texture and how well the ingredients complement each other. You can adjust the ingredient amounts based on the size of your platter and the number of guests you are serving.

 PREP TIME: 20 MINUTES
SERVES: 8 TO 10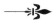

4 oz (100 g) hard salami
4 oz (100 g) good quality prosciutto, sliced thin
4 oz (100 g) mortadella, sliced
8 oz (250 g) soppresetta, sliced
12 oz (350 g) marinated artichokes heats, quartered
8 oz (250 g) roasted red peppers, thinly sliced
2 or 3 boiled eggs, chopped or sliced
4 oz (100 g) olives
4 oz (100 g) anchovies
Sea salt, to taste
½ cup (125 ml) extra-virgin olive oil
1 tablespoon balsamic vinegar

Arrange all ingredients decoratively on the platter, paying attention to contrasting colors, textures, and flavors.

Before serving, sprinkle the sea salt and drizzle the olive oil and balsamic vinegar over the ingredients.

ANTIPASTO OR ANTIPASTI?

I get this question all the time. Antipasto is singular, as in one antipasto platter; antipasti is plural— "appetizers." An antipasto platter, which is the traditional first course of a formal Italian meal, includes cured meats, olives, pepperoncini, mushrooms, anchovies, artichokes, cheeses and pickled vegetables, and is seasoned with olive oil and vinegar.

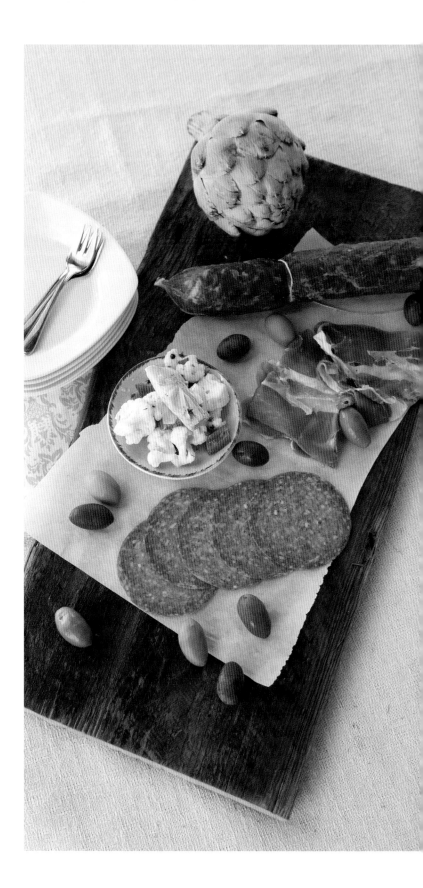

LAMB POPS WRAPPED WITH PROSCIUTTO

These quick, yet gourmet treats make an impressive appetizer for any occasion. You can assemble the chops in advance and keep them refrigerated until you're ready to cook them. If you can't find lamb chops, you can ask your butcher to cut up a rack of lamb into individual chops.

PREP TIME: 15 MINUTES
COOK TIME: 10 MINUTES
SERVES: 5 TO 6

12 lamb chops
2 teaspoons sea salt
1½ teaspoons freshly ground pepper
3 to 4 tablespoons (or more) olive oil
4 cloves garlic, minced
8 rosemary sprigs, removed from stem and chopped
12 slices thinly-cut prosciutto

Preheat oven to 150°F (65°C). Place a baking sheet in the oven.

Spread out the lamb chops on a clean work surface and season both sides with salt and pepper.

Combine the minced garlic and rosemary together on the work surface. Rub the garlic and rosemary mixture onto both sides of each lamb chop.

Wrap a slice of prosciutto around each chop.

Let rest while you heat a large skillet over medium-high heat. Once the pan is hot, add about 2 tablespoons of olive oil.

Place the 4 to 6 lamb chops in the pan and sauté for 3 to 4 minutes per side or until the prosciutto is browned. Place lamb chops in the oven to finish cooking and to keep them warm before serving.

CINDY'S NOTE

Here's a great way to mince garlic finely enough to use as a rub. Peel and coarsely chop the garlic cloves, then sprinkle a pinch of sea salt over the garlic. Use the flat of a chef's knife to press the garlic and salt into the board to make a paste.

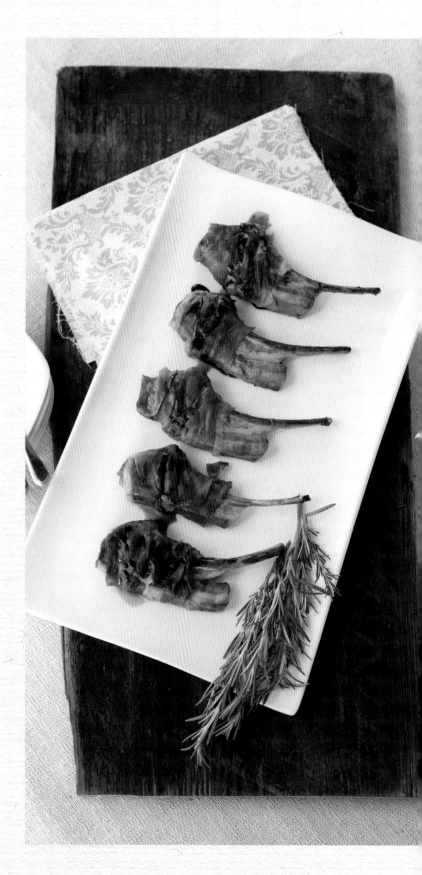

GRILLED ARTICHOKES WITH LEMON PESTO AIOLI

There's something special about starting out with whole, fresh artichokes and ending up with a delicious appetizer. I always prepare a few extra artichokes—one to enjoy right away and at least one to save for later.

 PREP TIME: 10 MINUTES
COOK TIME: 25 MINUTES
SERVES: 4

FOR THE ARTICHOKES

4 large fresh artichokes
¼ cup (30 g) almond meal
1 cup (45 g) Italian parsley, finely
  chopped
1 teaspoon dried basil
1 teaspoon dried thyme
1½ teaspoons sea salt, plus more
  for sprinkling
1 teaspoon freshly ground pepper
¼ teaspoon dried red pepper flakes
  (optional)
Juice of 1 lemon
3 cloves garlic, chopped
6 tablespoons olive oil, divided
1 teaspoon freshly ground black
  pepper

CINDY'S NOTE

The aioli can be prepared in advance, and the artichokes can be steamed earlier in the day, or even the day before. When you're ready to serve, just grill and enjoy!

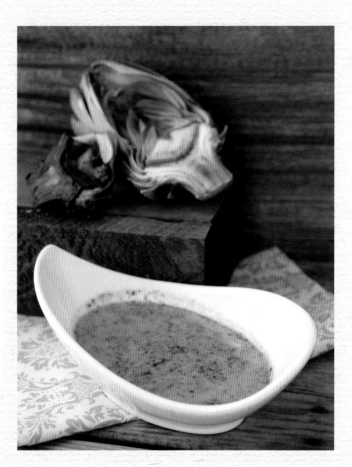

LEMON BASIL PESTO AIOLI

¼ cup (5 g) fresh basil leaves
¼ cup (25 g) walnuts, chopped or
  halved
2 cloves garlic, chopped
1 teaspoon sea salt
½ teaspoon freshly ground pepper
2 tablespoons fresh lemon juice
¼ cup (65 ml) extra-virgin olive oil
½ cup (125 ml) Paleo Mayonnaise
  (page 32)
3 tablespoons coconut oil or heavy
  coconut cream

PREPARING THE ARTICHOKES

Cut any torn leaves from the artichokes with kitchen scissors. With a knife, cut off about a third of the top of each artichoke and trim the stem. Smack the top of the artichoke against the counter or a wooden board.

In a medium mixing bowl, combine the almond meal, parsley, basil, thyme, salt, pepper, red pepper flakes (if using), lemon juice, garlic and 3 tablespoons of olive oil.

Fill a large pot with about four inches (10 cm) of water, or prepare a pot with a steamer basket.

Place the artichokes in the pot or steamer basket, then open the leaves and divide the parsley mixture into a few of the leaves. Drizzle two more tablespoons of the olive oil over them.

Place the pot over medium heat, cover and steam artichokes for 35 to 40 minutes. Check the water level every 15 minutes; add more if needed. To test the artichokes for doneness, gently pull on a leaf. If it comes out easily, the artichokes are done.

Remove artichokes from the pot and allow to cool for about 10 minutes. Preheat a grill or indoor grill pan.

Meanwhile, cut each artichoke in half lengthwise. Use a spoon to remove the fuzzy hair in the center, but do not touch the heart.

Brush each artichoke with the remaining olive oil and sprinkle a pinch of salt and pepper over the cut surface. Place cut side down on the heated grill or grill pan and cook for 5 to 7 minutes, until the lines from the grill are visible. Turn the artichokes over and grill for 1 minute more. Arrange on a platter.

MAKING THE LEMON BASIL PESTO AIOLI

Place the basil leaves, walnuts, garlic, salt, pepper, lemon juice and olive oil in a food processor. Pulse until smooth, then transfer to a decorative bowl. Mix in the mayonnaise and coconut oil or cream.

Serve alongside the platter of grilled artichokes.

GRILLED CALAMARI SALAD

I order this salad, an Italian favorite, whenever I find it on the menu at a restaurant in Tuscany. It's lovely with a glass of red wine before a main course. I've noticed that many Italian restaurants in the U.S. now offer a grilled calamari salad, adding their own twist.

 PREP TIME: 15 MINUTES
COOK TIME: 5 MINUTES
SERVES: 4

1 lb (500 g) fresh calamari

1 teaspoon sea salt

½ teaspoon freshly ground black pepper

4 tablespoons olive oil (divided)

Zest of 1 lemon

Juice of 1 lemon, (about 1 tablespoon)

½ cup (60 g) thinly sliced red onions

1 pepperoncini, cut into thin rings

2 tablespoons kalamata olives, pitted and halved

2 tablespoons capers

¼ cup (5 g) fresh parsley, chopped

Preheat a grill pan over medium-high heat.

Gently rinse the calamari and pat dry with a clean white kitchen towel. Season lightly with salt and pepper.

Add 2 tablespoons olive oil to the pan. Once the oil is hot, add the calamari and grill for 2 minutes on each side. Remove from pan and slice into thin rings.

Combine the remaining 2 tablespoons olive oil, lemon zest, lemon juice, red onions, pepperoncini, olives, capers and fresh parsley in a large bowl. Add the calamari rings.

Toss together and enjoy!

CINDY'S NOTE
This recipe should be served and enjoyed immediately after it's prepared.

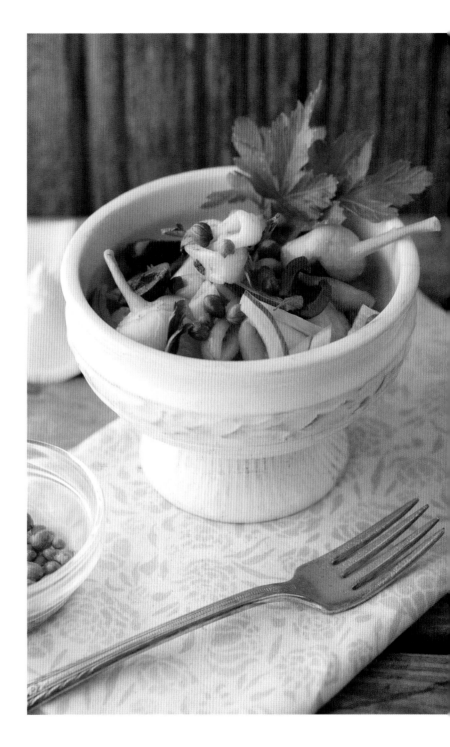

TUSCAN MUSHROOMS

This appetizer is often served in Italian homes, including my own. The baked mushrooms are flavorful and satisfying, but not too filling, so they're a great starter for a fancy meal.

 PREP TIME: 15 MINUTES
COOK TIME: 20 MINUTES
SERVES: 6

1 lb (500 g) large white button mushrooms, cleaned, stems removed
3 tablespoons extra-virgin olive oil, divided
1½ teaspoons sea salt, divided
1 teaspoon freshly ground black pepper, divided
½ cup (70 g) diced roasted red bell peppers
½ cup (70 g) pitted and diced green olives
2 green onions (scallions) green and white parts, sliced
¼ cup (5 g) finely chopped fresh basil leaves

Preheat the oven to 400°F (200°C).

Place the mushrooms in a medium bowl and add 2 tablespoons of the olive oil. Season with 1 teaspoon of the sea salt and ½ teaspoon of the pepper, then stir together gently.

Combine the roasted red peppers, olives and green onions in a small bowl. Add the remaining 1 tablespoon of the olive oil and the remaining ½ teaspoon sea salt and ½ teaspoon pepper, then stir to coat.

Place the mushrooms, cavity side up, on a parchment paper-lined baking sheet. Spoon the red pepper filling into each mushroom cap. Bake until the mushrooms are tender, about 20 minutes.

Transfer the mushrooms to a serving platter, sprinkle with chopped basil, and serve.

CINDY'S NOTE
I don't like to waste food, and I find it's easy to use leftovers, or parts of them, to create a totally new meal. Leftover Tuscan Mushrooms are fantastic sautéed with chicken or added to a sauce or breakfast frittata.

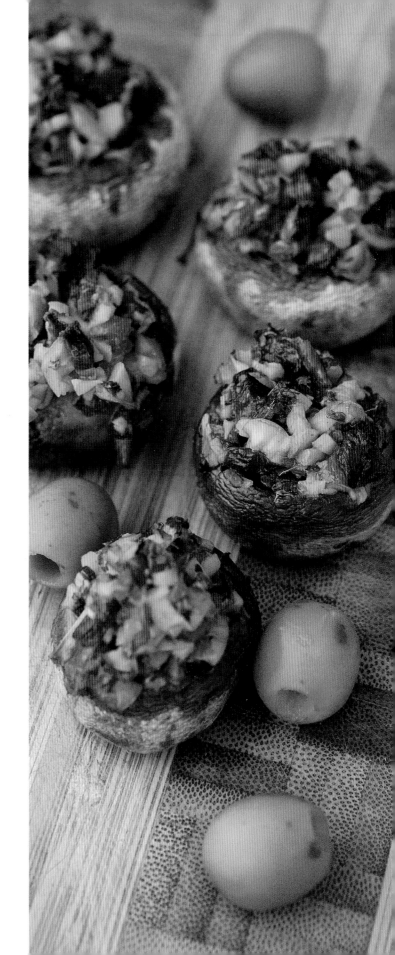

PROSCIUTTO-WRAPPED GOAT CHEESE & FIGS

These will wow your guests with their beauty, but the big smiles will come after the first bite. The sweetness of the fig with the melted goat cheese and the barely crisp prosciutto makes a fabulous combination.

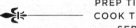

PREP TIME: 20 MINUTES
COOK TIME: 10 MINUTES
SERVES: 2 TO 4

6 whole fresh figs, cut in half lengthwise

3 tablespoons balsamic vinegar

4 oz (100 g) goat cheese

6 slices prosciutto, halved

2 to 3 tablespoons raw honey (preferably local)

2 cups (60 g) washed baby arugula

2 to 3 tablespoons extra-virgin olive oil

Sea salt, to taste

Preheat oven to 400°F (200°C). Line a baking sheet with parchment paper and place fig halves on the sheet, spacing evenly.

Pour a little balsamic vinegar over each fig half, then fill each center with goat cheese.

Wrap each fig half with a slice of prosciutto, then drizzle each one with honey.

Place in oven on the top rack for 8 to 10 minutes.

Spread the arugula over a serving platter or shallow dish. Remove the figs from the oven and arrange them on the bed of arugula. Drizzle extra-virgin olive oil over, and sprinkle with sea salt.

Serve immediately.

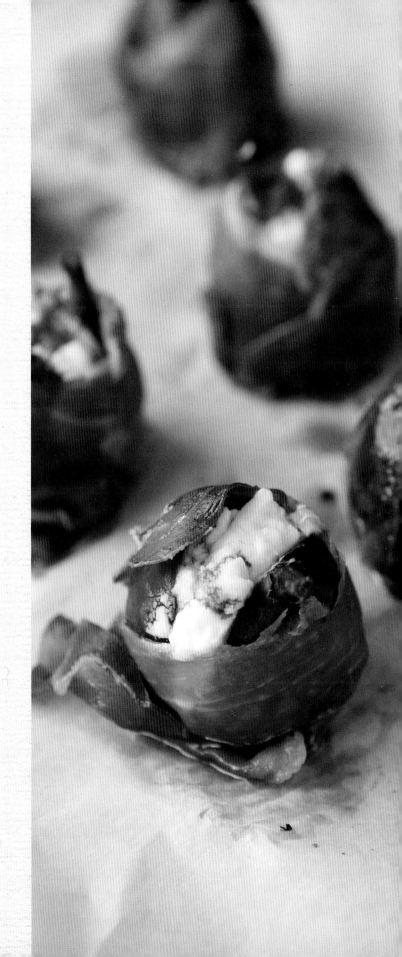

SEVEN-LAYER DEVILED EGG DIP

When I see people eating deviled eggs at parties, they always look so happy as they pop them into their mouths. This recipe is a layered version of the favorite standby. I love to serve this in a trifle dish—it looks so pretty!

PREP TIME: 20 MINUTES
COOK TIME: 12 MINUTES
SERVES: 6

5 large eggs

½ cup (40 g) romaine lettuce, shredded

2 celery stalks, thinly sliced

3 green onions (scallions), green and white parts, chopped

4 oz (70 g) cherry tomatoes, sliced in half

2 teaspoons sea salt, divided

1 teaspoon freshly ground black pepper, divided

1 cup (250 g) Paleo Mayonnaise (page 32)

1 small red onion, finely chopped

3 tablespoons chopped fresh parsley

1¼ teaspoons Dijon mustard

1 teaspoon paprika

3 tablespoons chopped dill

½ cup (100 g) pickles, sliced

2 avocados, peeled and chopped

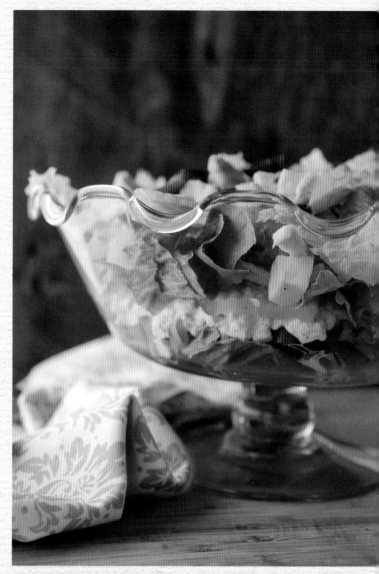

Place the eggs in a single layer in a saucepan and cover with 1 to 1½ in (2.5 to 4 cm) cold water.

With the pan uncovered, bring the water to a boil, then cover. Let boil for 30 seconds, then remove from heat, still covered, and allow to stand for 12 minutes. Remove the eggs from the pan with a slotted spoon and place in a bowl to cool.

Make the first layer by laying half the romaine at the bottom of the bowl, then add the celery and green onions.

Next, use half the tomatoes to make the next layer. Sprinkle about 1 teaspoon of sea salt and ½ teaspoon or more freshly ground pepper over top.

Peel and chop the cooked eggs and put them in a separate mixing bowl. Add the mayonnaise, red onion, parsley, mustard, paprika, dill, remaining 1 teaspoon sea salt and remaining ½ teaspoon freshly ground pepper. Stir to combine well.

Make the next layer with the eggs, using all the egg mixture.

Add a layer of sliced pickles.

Add a second layer of romaine, using the rest of the lettuce.

Add a second layer of tomatoes, using the rest of the tomatoes.

Cover and refrigerate for at least 1 hour. When ready to serve, top with the chopped avocados.

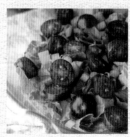

Make the first layer with half the lettuce, the celery, and the green onions. Use half the tomatoes to make a second layer.

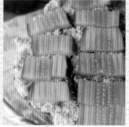

Add the prepared egg mixture, and top with the sliced pickles.

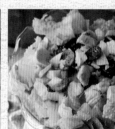

Add the remaining lettuce. Make the final layer with the remaining tomatoes and top with chopped avocado.

GRILLED WHITE ANCHOVIES WITH GREMOLATA

What's gremolata? It sounds kind of sexy and sophisticated, but it's a deceptively simple condiment made from finely minced parsley, minced garlic and lemon zest. It's traditionally served with osso buco, but it goes beautifully with steak, chicken or seafood. You can also substitute mint for the parsley and serve it with lamb chops. Anchovies are a favorite in Italy. Grilled white anchovies are one of my favorite starters to enjoy with wine in the afternoon when I'm in Tuscany. Fresh sardines can also be used in this recipe, but white anchovies are superior if you can get them.

 PREP TIME: 15 MINUTES
COOK TIME: 10 MINUTES
SERVES: 4

FOR THE WHITE ANCHOVIES

1 lb (500 g) white anchovies, scaled and cleaned

1 tablespoon olive oil

1 teaspoon sea salt

½ teaspoon freshly ground black pepper

FOR THE GREMOLATA

Zest of 1 lemon

¼ cup (5 g) fresh parsley, finely chopped

3 cloves garlic, minced

¾ teaspoon sea salt

¼ teaspoon freshly ground black pepper

2 to 3 tablespoons extra-virgin olive oil

Rinse the anchovies and pat dry, then place them on a plate. Drizzle the olive oil over top and season with salt and pepper.

Combine the lemon zest, parsley, garlic, salt and pepper in a mixing bowl. Whisk in the olive oil and set aside.

Preheat a grill pan over medium-high heat. Brush the pan with a little olive oil, and then place the anchovies on the grill. Cook for 5 minutes per side. Be very careful when turning the fish over halfway through grilling—they are quite delicate.

Remove from heat and arrange on a serving platter. Spoon the gremolata over the anchovies and serve immediately.

> ### CINDY'S NOTE
> To make really flavorful lemon zest, use a vegetable peeler to remove the rind from a lemon rather than using a grater. Chop the resulting strip of peel finely. The chopped peel from half a lemon makes about 2 teaspoons of lemon zest.

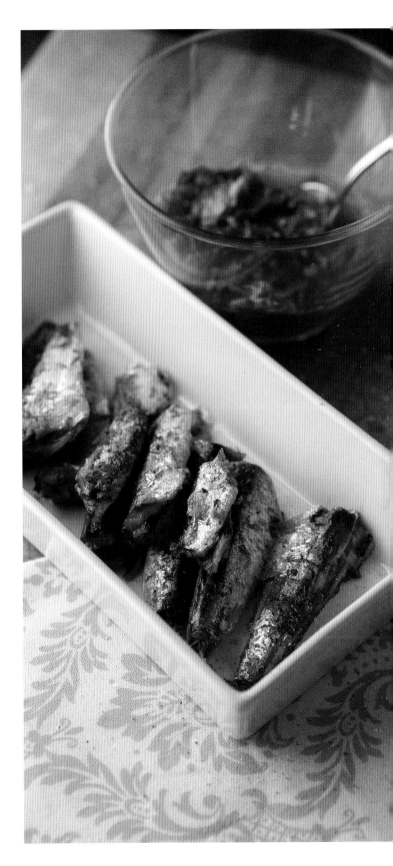

ROASTED BEET SALAD WITH DIJON SHALLOTS

Beets have become very popular lately, with beet salads appearing on many restaurant menus. It makes me so happy when I visit a friend's house and they ask me, "Do you like beets?" I remember eating tasteless, mushy canned beets as a little girl, and not enjoying them much. Roasted beets are a completely different proposition—lively and full of flavor. The Dijon dressing elevates them from tasty to extraordinary.

If you're already using your oven for something else, why not pop a few beets in there to roast for this salad? If you keep a well-stocked pantry, you should have all of the other ingredients handy.

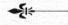 PREP TIME: 15 MINUTES
COOK TIME: 1 HOUR
SERVES: 6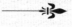

1 bunch medium beets

1 tablespoon olive oil

2 teaspoons sea salt

3 cups (100 g) mixed greens (frisée, mesclun, or other greens)

3 oz (75 g) goat cheese

½ cup (64 g) walnuts, chopped

FOR THE VINAIGRETTE

1½ tablespoons minced shallot

1 tablespoon Dijon mustard

3 tablespoons red wine vinegar

2 tablespoons raw honey (preferably local)

¾ teaspoon sea salt

½ teaspoon freshly ground black pepper

½ cup (125 ml) extra-virgin olive oil

CINDY'S NOTE

How can you avoid staining your fingers red when you prepare fresh beets? I cut the greens off as closely as possible, then scrub the beet with a brush under running water to really get it clean. After roasting, the skin should come off very easily. If you work fast, your fingers don't get stained; you can also wear gloves. Or you can try peeling the beet under cold running water.

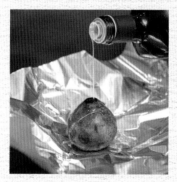

Place a washed and trimmed beet in the foil cup and drizzle with olive oil.

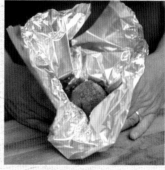

Sprinkle on some salt and gather the foil around each beet before baking.

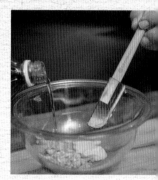

Whisk the vinaigrette ingredients when adding the olive oil.

Preheat oven to 400°F (200°C). Have a baking sheet ready.

Scrub the beets and trim the stems to the top of the beet.

Make a cup from a piece of aluminum foil and place one beet inside. Drizzle a little olive oil over the beet and sprinkle some sea salt on top, then seal the foil at the top and place on the baking sheet. Repeat for the remaining beets.

Roast the beets for one hour. Test for doneness with a knife; it should pierce the beet easily. Remove from oven and allow to cool enough to handle.

Use your hands or a paring knife to peel the skin from the beets. It should be easy to remove.

Slice or chop the beets and set aside.

Arrange the greens on a large bowl or platter. Top with spoonfuls of the goat cheese and the walnuts, and spread the beets over.

To make the vinaigrette, whisk together the shallots, Dijon mustard, red wine vinegar, honey, salt and pepper in a small bowl. Add the olive oil in a steady stream as you continue whisking.

Pour the dressing over the salad and serve.

ITALIAN CHOPPED SALAD

When you say the words "Italian Chopped Salad," everyone gets excited. You can add any or all of your favorite Italian ingredients. Sometimes I throw in just about everything in my pantry or refrigerator. If something sounds appealing, use it!

PREP TIME: 20 MINUTES
SERVES: 6

1 clove garlic, crushed

2 tablespoons red wine vinegar

1 teaspoon dried oregano

½ teaspoon sea salt

½ teaspoon freshly ground black pepper

¼ cup (60 ml) extra-virgin olive oil

2 large romaine hearts, chopped

1 small head radicchio, chopped

One 14-oz (400-g) can quartered artichoke hearts, drained

One 14-oz (400-g) can hearts of palm, drained and sliced

1 tender celery rib, thinly sliced

½ small red onion, thinly sliced

1 cup (200 g) cherry tomatoes

½ cup (100 g) pitted green olives, preferably Sicilian

Anchovies, (optional)

8 to 10 slices hard salami, rolled into cylinders

In a mixing bowl, whisk together the garlic, red wine vinegar, oregano, and salt and pepper. Continue whisking while pouring in the olive oil. Set aside.

Layer the romaine hearts and radicchio to cover the bottom of a large serving platter.

Spread the artichoke hearts, hearts of palm, celery, red onion, cherry tomatoes and olives on top of the greens.

Place the anchovies, if using, in the center of the salad. Arrange the salami rolls around the edges of the platter.

Pour the dressing over the salad just before serving.

CINDY'S NOTE

For a perfect lunch, top this salad with last night's protein, or grill some eggplant slices and season them with balsamic vinegar. Canned tuna or smoked salmon are also good additions to this salad.

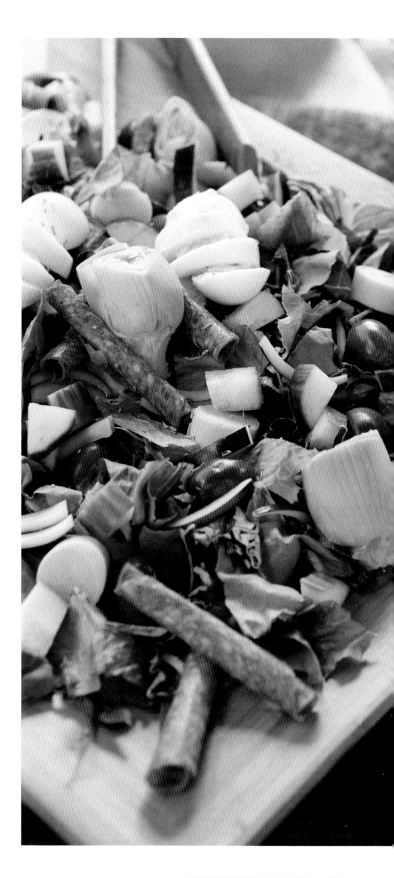

SPINACH & SMOKED SALMON SALAD WITH LEMON DILL DRESSING

Because my husband and I are a very social couple, we frequently throw last-minute dinner parties. In one case, we invited some friends on the spur of the moment, and I hadn't gone shopping for a while. Luckily, I had all of the ingredients on hand to create this delicious salad. It looks gourmet, but takes only a few minutes to prepare!

 **PREP TIME: 15 MINUTES
SERVES: 4**

3 tablespoons extra-virgin olive oil

2 tablespoons fresh lemon juice

2 tablespoons fresh dill, chopped

1 teaspoon sea salt

¾ teaspoon freshly ground black pepper

6 to 8 cups (200 to 250 g) baby spinach

6 oz (170 g) thinly sliced smoked salmon,
  cut crosswise into ½-inch (1.25-cm) strips

1 medium English cucumber, peeled, halved
  lengthwise, and thinly sliced

2 green onions (scallions), thinly sliced

In a large bowl, whisk together the olive oil, lemon juice, dill, salt and pepper until well blended.

Add the spinach, smoked salmon, cucumber and green onions to the bowl and toss well.

Transfer the salad to plates and serve.

CINDY'S NOTE

If smoked salmon is on sale at your local fish market, pick up a little extra to freeze for later. It thaws quickly and adds a special touch even when you're short on time.

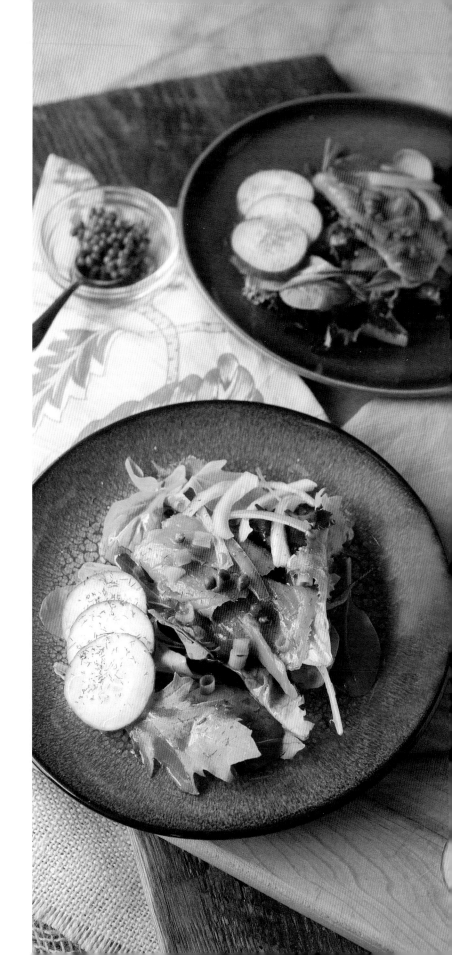

ITALIAN-STYLE TOMATO SALAD

This was Nana's favorite salad. I remember her always asking me, "Do you want a tomato salad for lunch?" I miss her so much, and I treasure all the memories of our time together. This salad, with its aromatic basil and tangy dressing, evokes her presence in a single bite.

 PREP TIME: 15 MINUTES
SERVES: 4

¼ cup (60 ml) extra-virgin olive oil

1 tablespoon red wine vinegar

1 teaspoon sea salt

1 teaspoon minced shallots

4 plum tomatoes, chopped

½ cup (75 g) thinly sliced cucumber

1 small red onion, thinly sliced

⅓ cup (10 g) fresh basil leaves, chopped

1 tablespoon capers, drained

Whisk the olive oil, vinegar, salt and shallots together in a medium bowl.

Add the plum tomatoes, cucumbers, red onion, basil leaves and capers. Stir gently to combine all ingredients.

Transfer the salad a serving platter or bowl, and enjoy.

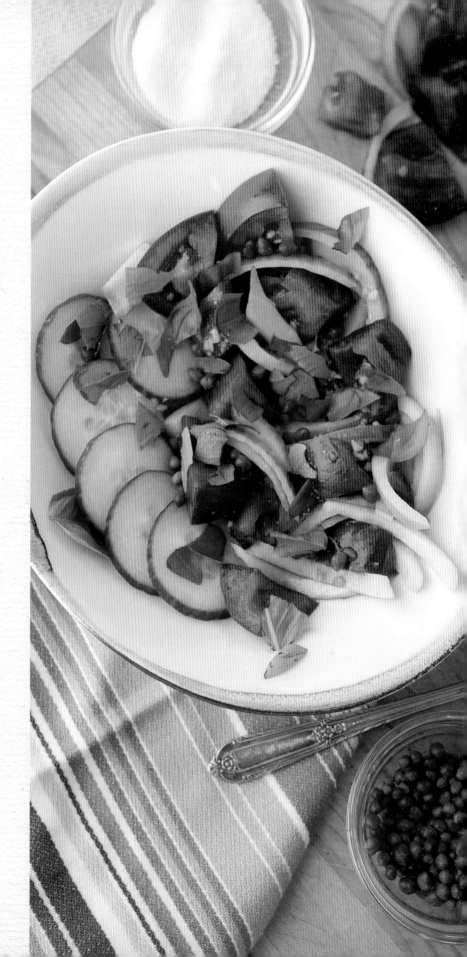

BABY KALE & MIXED GREENS SALAD WITH SHRIMP

Using baby kale makes a wonderfully delicate salad. The perfect dish for a break in the middle of the day!

 PREP TIME: 15 MINUTES
SERVES: 4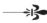

3 cups (125 g) baby kale
2 cups (85 g) mixed greens
1 cup (100 g) fresh mushrooms, sliced
1½ cups (150 g) cooked shrimp
1 avocado, sliced
1 teaspoon Dijon mustard
½ teaspoon sea salt
½ teaspoon freshly ground black pepper
1 tablespoon fresh lemon juice
½ cup (125 ml) extra-virgin olive oil

Spread out the baby kale and greens on a serving platter or shallow dish. Top with the mushrooms, shrimp and avocado slices.

In a small bowl, whisk together the mustard, salt, pepper, lemon juice and olive oil. Pour over the salad, toss and enjoy!

CINDY'S NOTES

When you find cooked frozen shrimp on sale, be sure to grab a bag. They thaw out fast and go well on salads.

Here are two ways to cook shelled and deveined fresh shrimp for a salad:

Sauté—Preheat a skillet over medium-high heat. Add coconut oil or unsalted butter; once hot, add shrimp to the pan. Cook large shrimp cook for 3 to 4 minutes, medium shrimp for 2½ to 3 minutes, and small or bay shrimp for 2 to 2½ minutes.

Boil—Fill a pot halfway with water and bring to a boil over high heat. Lower the heat to medium-high and add the shrimp. Cooking times are the same as for sautéing. Drain the shrimp and let cool.

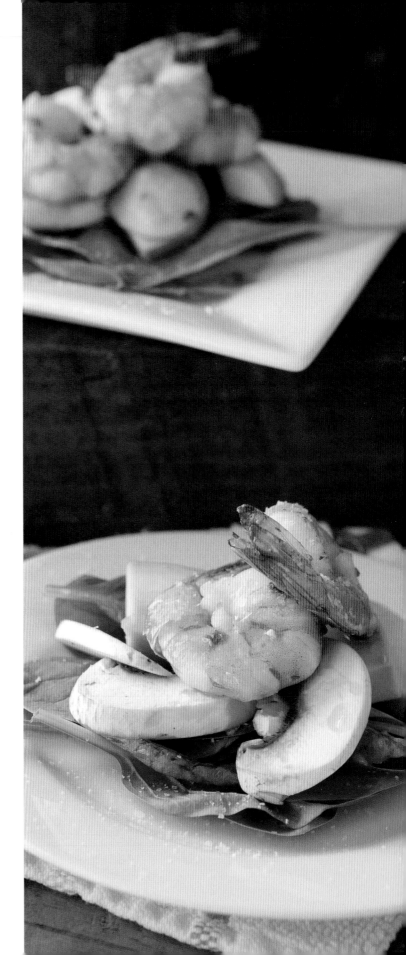

TUSCAN SEAFOOD SALAD

One of the best things about the markets in Tuscany is that you can peruse the fresh salads and meats available, order what you want, and have it right there with a glass of wine. This recipe is similar to an especially memorable salad I enjoyed at the market one day. The flavors of the seafood mingled together make it a perfect midday salad.

**PREP TIME: 15 MINUTES, PLUS
30 MINUTES FOR REFRIGERATION
COOK TIME: 5 MINUTES
SERVES: 4**

2 tablespoons olive oil
½ lb (225 g) sea scallops
¼ lb (125 g) medium shrimp
¼ lb (125 g) calamari rings
2 cloves garlic, minced
½ cup (70 g) small capers
Juice of 1 lemon
1 small red onion, thinly sliced

⅓ cup (80 ml) extra-virgin olive oil, plus more for drizzling
1 tablespoon fresh parsley, finely chopped
1 tablespoon fresh chives, chopped
1½ teaspoons sea salt
¾ teaspoon freshly ground black pepper
1 lemon, quartered, to serve with salad

Place a large skillet over medium-high heat and add the olive oil. Once hot, add the scallops, shrimp and calamari rings. Cook, stirring, for about 4 minutes, then remove from the heat.

Add the garlic to the pan and stir with a spatula to mix thoroughly with the oil and seafood. Allow to stand for 1 minute, then transfer to a large bowl or platter.

Add the capers, lemon juice, red onion, extra-virgin olive oil, parsley and chives, then the salt and pepper. Stir well to combine, then cover. Refrigerate for 30 minutes before serving.

When ready to serve, distribute among 4 bowls. Place a lemon quarter on the side and drizzle the salad with extra-virgin olive oil.

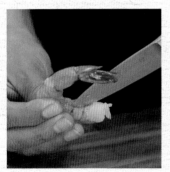

Remove the shrimp legs and shells, leaving on the tail intact. Devein the shrimp.

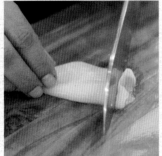

Slice the calamari into rings.

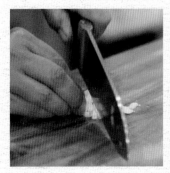

Mince the garlic.

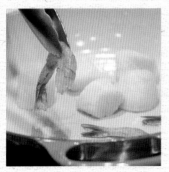

Cook the seafood before adding the garlic and proceeding with the rest of the recipe.

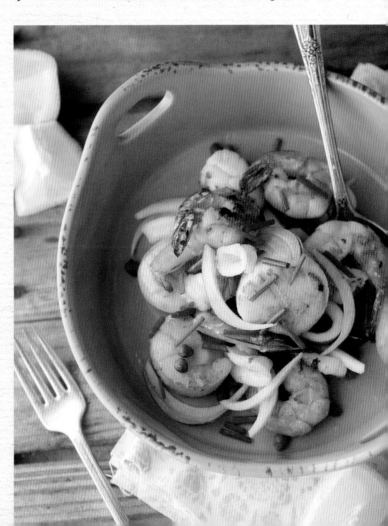

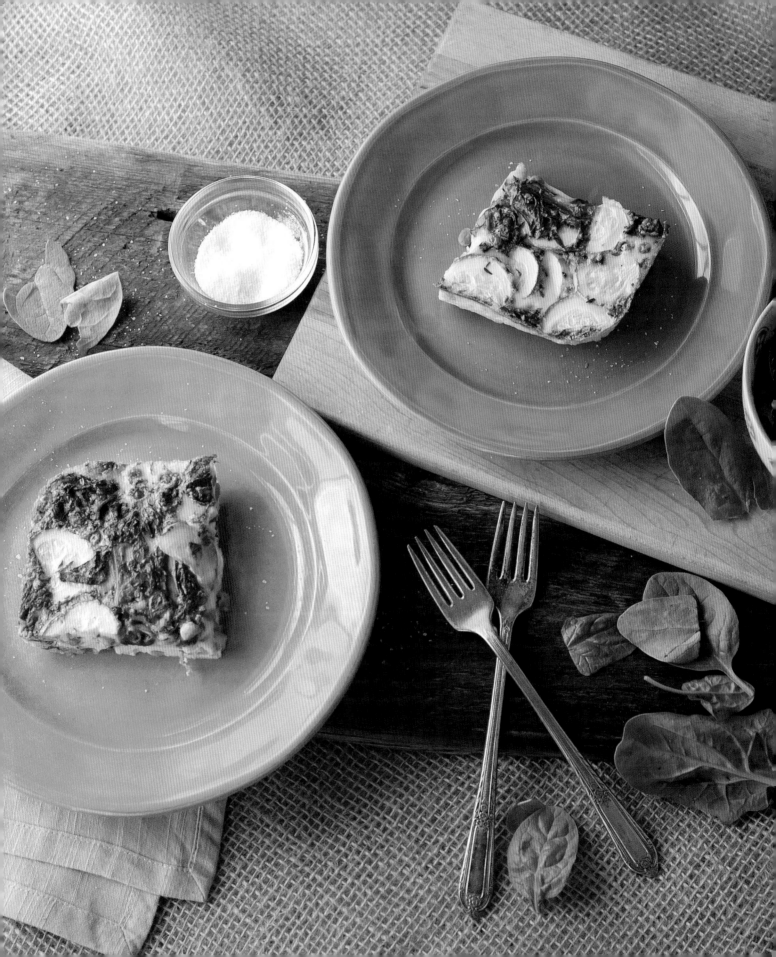

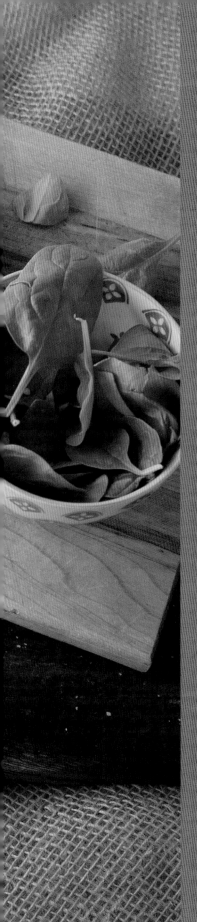

BRUNCH

Every meal is gratifying when your family is sitting at the table talking together, but brunch is always special. I remember Nana filling the table with a variety of brunch choices, fruits and grilled vegetables. Converting her dishes to Paleo standards was actually easy. I don't feel that anything was lost—in fact, it has actually added flavor to the original recipes.

I really can't choose a favorite brunch recipe. I love them all and enjoy them frequently. When we have guests from out of town, I often make a few different brunch dishes, so we can all have several items to choose from.

I hope these recipes evoke the feeling of sitting at a little café in Tuscany with a cappuccino or espresso. I love how Italians yell at each other and wave their hands up and down with so much energy and passion. We also cook this way, and we love nothing more than for you to eat! Don't ever upset an Italian by turning them down when they offer you food. Just sit down and enjoy.

SCRAMBLED EGGS WITH SMOKED SALMON & ARUGULA

I often make this easy dish for a crowd. My husband and I entertain often, and I'd rather spend time with my guests than stand over the stove. The vibrant colors and flavors of this dish are a great eye-opener, and the peppery arugula really brings it to life.

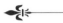 PREP TIME: 10 MINUTES
COOK TIME: 10 MINUTES
SERVES: 4

8 slices smoked salmon

12 large eggs

¼ cup (65 ml) canned coconut milk

1 teaspoon sea salt

½ teaspoon freshly ground black pepper

2 tablespoons coconut oil or ghee

2 cups (60 g) washed arugula

Coarsely chop the smoked salmon, then set aside.

In a large mixing bowl whisk the eggs, then add the coconut milk, salt and pepper. Whisk to combine, then add the salmon.

Place a large skillet over medium heat. Add the coconut oil or ghee.

When the oil or ghee is hot, pour in the egg mixture and cook for about 1 minute, then stir with a wooden spoon. Allow to cook for 3 minutes more, then add the arugula and stir. Continue to cook until the eggs begin to set but are still moist, about 5 to 7 minutes. (They will continue cooking after the pan is removed from the heat).

To serve, just bring the pan to the table and have everyone dig in!

CINDY'S NOTE

Prepackaged smoked salmon is available just about everywhere. I find, however, that I can get the best and freshest smoked salmon at my local fish market.

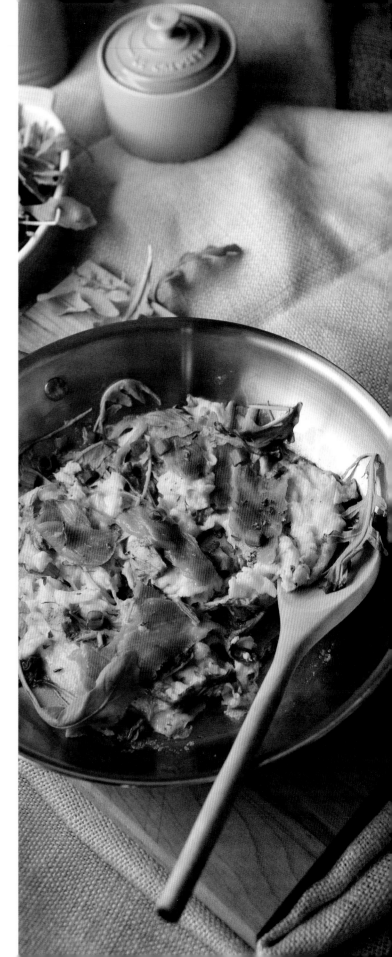

EGGS IN PURGATORY

Nana used to ask us if we wanted uova in purgatorio *for breakfast in the morning—so called because the spicy tomato sauce makes the eggs hot as hell. This makes a good weekend breakfast: you prepare the whole dish in one pan, bring it to the table, and let everyone help themselves.*

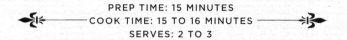

PREP TIME: 15 MINUTES
COOK TIME: 15 TO 16 MINUTES
SERVES: 2 TO 3

2 tablespoons olive oil

½ small yellow onion, finely chopped

1 large zucchini, sliced

4 baby bella or cremini mushrooms, sliced

2 cloves garlic, minced

½ teaspoon dried red pepper flakes

1 teaspoon dried basil

1 teaspoon dried oregano

1 teaspoon dried parsley

¾ teaspoon sea salt

¼ teaspoon freshly ground black pepper

One 14-oz (500-g) can crushed or petite diced tomatoes

4 to 6 large eggs

Fresh herbs for garnish

Preheat oven to 375°F (150°C).

Place a large oven-safe skillet over medium heat. Add the oil.

When the oil is very hot add the onion, zucchini, mushrooms and garlic. Cook for about 3 minutes, stirring with a wooden spoon.

Add the red pepper flakes, basil, oregano, parsley, salt and pepper. Stir to combine.

Add tomatoes and bring to a boil. Taste sauce and adjust seasonings if necessary.

Carefully crack the eggs one at a time into the sauce, leaving space between each egg.

Bake in oven until the whites are set but the yolks are still runny, about 11 or 12 minutes. Top with fresh herbs.

Scoop out an egg along with vegetables and sauce for each serving.

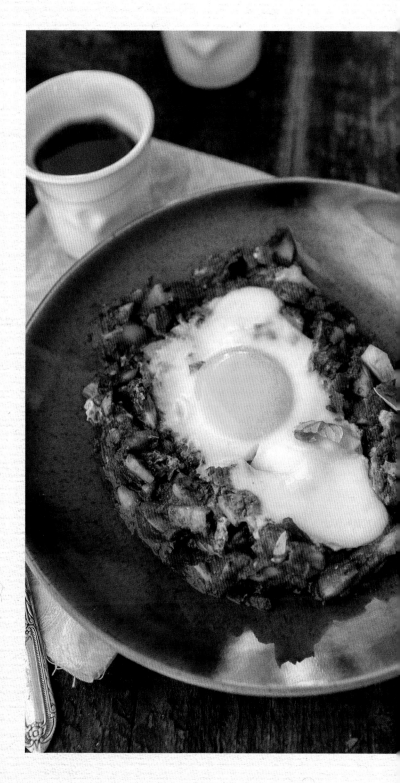

TUSCAN VEGETABLE & HERB BAKED OMELET

This omelet makes a lovely Saturday breakfast for family or overnight guests. You can prepare the ingredients the night before; in the morning, just put it in the oven, get the coffee going and set the table.

Since any cooked protein goes well in this frittata, it's a great way to use up leftovers from the week. Served with a side salad, it also makes a nice light dinner.

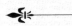

PREP TIME: 20 MINUTES
COOK TIME: 30 MINUTES
SERVES: 6

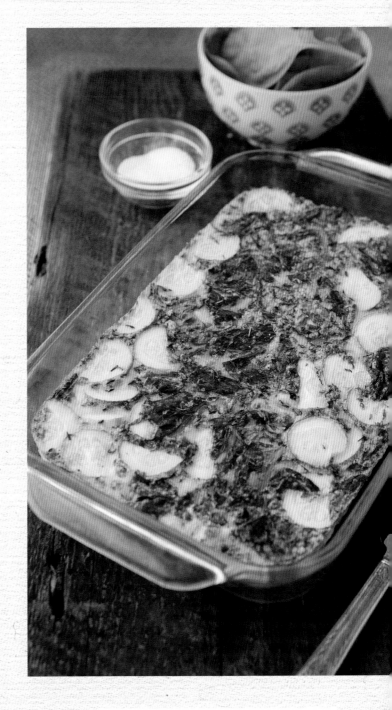

12 large eggs

2 tablespoons water

1 teaspoon sea salt

¾ teaspoon freshly ground black pepper

1 teaspoon dried basil

2 tablespoons olive oil or coconut oil, plus more for coating pan

1 small zucchini, sliced thin

2 cloves garlic, minced (about 2 teaspoons)

2 green onions (scallions) green and white parts, sliced (reserve some for garnish)

⅓ cup (40 g) frozen petite peas, thawed

1 cup (30 g) fresh spinach

1 teaspoon fresh thyme, chopped (reserve some for garnish)

2 tablespoons fresh parsley, chopped (reserve some for garnish)

Preheat oven to 350°F (175°C).

Whisk together the eggs, water, salt, pepper and basil in a large bowl. Set aside.

Heat a large skillet over medium heat, then add the oil. Once hot, add the zucchini and cook for 3 to 5 minutes, stirring or tossing once. Add the garlic and sliced green onions and cook for 1 minute more. Remove from heat and let cool.

Add the peas, spinach, fresh thyme and parsley to the egg mixture and stir. Add the cooked zucchini, garlic and green onions, and stir to combine all ingredients.

Brush a 9 x 13-inch (23 x 33-cm) baking pan with oil or butter.

Pour the egg mixture into the baking pan. Bake for 25 to 30 minutes, or until the center is firm.

Top with the reserved sliced green onions and fresh thyme and parsley.

CINDY'S NOTE
The fresh herbs really make this dish but if you only have dried herbs to top the omelet, you can use 1 teaspoon dried thyme and 2 teaspoons dried parsley.

ITALIAN BAKED EGGS

Nana and I loved making Italian baked eggs on the weekends, because we could prepare everyone's eggs the way they liked them best. Nana and I liked green onions on our baked eggs, while my grandfather preferred diced onions on his. Everyone had their own special request. We'd send my grandfather out to pick fresh tomatoes for us from his garden. If you can get fresh-picked tomatoes, this is a great way to enjoy them!

 PREP TIME: 15 MINUTES
COOK TIME: 20 MINUTES
SERVES: 4

½ tablespoon coconut oil, melted

2 tablespoons olive oil

1 shallot, finely chopped

2 cloves garlic, finely chopped

¼ teaspoon dried red pepper flakes (optional)

12 cherry tomatoes or 5 plum tomatoes, seeded and
  roughly chopped

1 tablespoon tomato paste

¾ teaspoon sea salt

½ teaspoon freshly ground black pepper

4 slices good-quality prosciutto (or 8 slices of bacon)

4 large eggs

Fresh herbs for garnish

Preheat the oven to 375°F (150°C).

Brush four 5-inch (12.5-cm) oven-safe ramekins with melted coconut oil.

Place a medium skillet over medium-high heat. Add the olive oil. When hot, add the shallot and garlic and sauté, stirring, until fragrant; about 3 minutes.

Stir in the red pepper flakes (if using), tomatoes and tomato paste. Cook until the sauce thickens, about 5 minutes. Season with salt and pepper.

Line each ramekin with a slice of prosciutto. Ladle a fourth of the tomato mixture into each one. Crack an egg into each ramekin.

Carefully place the ramekins on a baking sheet. Bake until the eggs are set, about 12 to 15 minutes.

Remove the ramekins from the oven and garnish with fresh herbs.

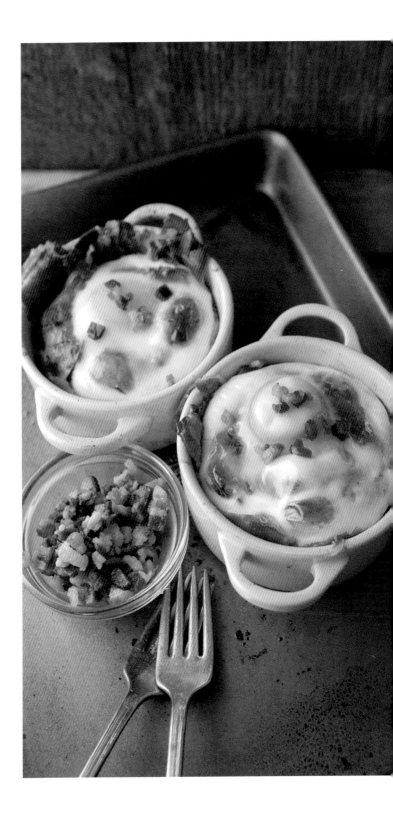

SPINACH & ARTICHOKE ROLLS

This recipe was inspired by my love of artichokes. These rolls just came together as I was creating this cookbook; they weren't on the original recipe list! I was very surprised that they turned out so well; the first bite was breathtaking. Go ahead and make these, but beware—it's hard to stop eating them!

PREP TIME: 30 TO 40 MINUTES,
NOT INCLUDING REFRIGERATION TIME
COOK TIME: 25 MINUTES
SERVES: 6

FOR THE DOUGH

2½ cups (250 g) blanched almond flour, plus extra for
  the work surface
¼ cup (30 g) coconut flour
¼ cup (30 g) tapioca flour, plus extra for the work surface
2 tablespoons coconut sugar
½ teaspoon baking soda
1 teaspoon sea salt
3 large eggs, at room temperature
¼ cup (65 ml) melted coconut oil, plus extra for coating tins

FOR THE FILLING

One 12-oz (340-g) can artichokes, drained and
  roughly chopped
One 10-oz (285-g) box frozen spinach, thawed
4 cloves garlic, peeled and chopped
½ teaspoon dried red pepper flakes
1 teaspoon dried basil
1 teaspoon dried thyme
1 teaspoon sea salt
½ teaspoon freshly ground black pepper
2 tablespoons olive oil or melted coconut oil
1 large egg

Preheat the oven to 350°F (175°C).

In a large mixing bowl, combine the almond flour, coconut flour, tapioca flour, coconut sugar, baking soda and salt and blend together with a fork.

Whisk the eggs in a separate small mixing bowl, then add the coconut oil and whisk again. Pour egg mixture into the dry ingredients and stir together using a spatula.

Form the dough into a disk, then wrap in waxed paper and refrigerate for 30 minutes.

Meanwhile, make the filling. Combine the artichokes, spinach, garlic, red pepper flakes, basil, thyme, salt and pepper in a food processor. Pulse until smooth.

Brush a 6-cup muffin tin with melted coconut oil.

Mix a small amount of almond meal and tapioca flour together and spread over a clean work surface. Roll the dough into an oblong shape about ¼ in (6 mm) thick, adding more almond-tapioca flour as needed.

Brush the rolled-out dough with olive oil or melted coconut oil. Spread the artichoke mixture on the dough in an even layer to about ¼ in (6 mm) from the top edge.

Starting at the bottom, roll the dough tightly to the top edge, sealing to make a log. Cut into 6 even pieces, then place the resulting rolls in the greased muffin tin, pressing them gently into place.

Whisk the egg in a small bowl. Brush the surface of each roll with beaten egg.

Bake the rolls for 18 to 20 minutes or until brown. Remove them from the muffin tin and let them cool slightly before enjoying them.

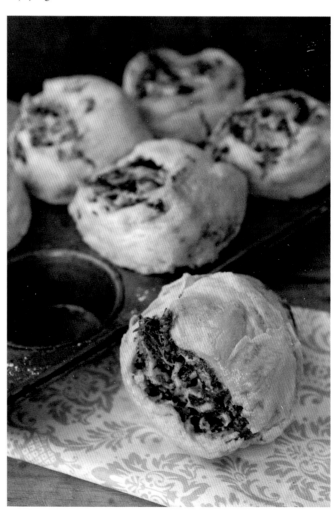

MEATY ITALIAN FRITTATA

A frittata is an Italian-style omelet that is normally partly cooked on the stove in a cast-iron pan, then finished in the oven. It's served in wedges straight from the pan. A frittata is a great use for your favorite meat and vegetables, and you can incorporate leftovers for a one-of-a-kind version. You can even top it with leftover "Sunday sauce" (a slow-cooked Italian tomato sauce that's loaded with meat).

PREP TIME: 15 MINUTES
COOK TIME: 20 MINUTES
SERVES: 4

8 large eggs

¼ cup (65 ml) coconut milk

2 green onions (scallions), white and green parts, sliced

1½ teaspoons sea salt

1 teaspoon freshly ground black pepper

3 tablespoons coconut oil or olive oil, divided

2 mild pork or chicken sausages, casings removed

½ lb (250 g) ground beef or chicken

8 oz (250 g) cremini mushrooms, sliced

1 clove garlic, minced

1 red bell pepper, chopped

1 teaspoon dried basil

1 teaspoon dried parsley

½ teaspoon dried thyme

Preheat oven to 350°F (175°C).

In a large mixing bowl, whisk the eggs, coconut milk, sliced green onions, salt and pepper. Set aside.

Heat 1 tablespoon of the oil in a skillet over medium heat. Once hot, add the sausage and ground meat. Break apart using a wooden spoon and cook until well browned, about 10 minutes.

Add the mushrooms, and let cook for 2 minutes. Then add the garlic and red bell pepper. Continue to cook for about 3 minutes, then remove from heat and allow to cool.

Add the egg mixture to the cooled meat and vegetables and stir to combine well. Add the basil, parsley and thyme, and mix again.

Brush a baking dish with the remaining 2 tablespoons of oil. Pour in the egg and meat mixture. Bake for 20 minutes, or until a knife comes out clean when inserted in the middle.

Allow to rest for 5 minutes after removing from oven, then slice and serve!

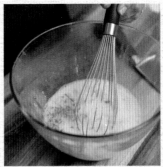

Whisk the eggs in a large bowl and add coconut milk and sliced green onions to the egg mixture. Set aside.

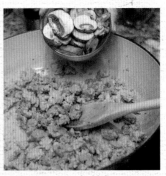

Brown the meat and add the mushrooms and garlic.

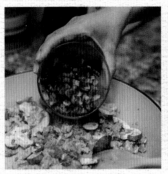

Add the bell peppers.

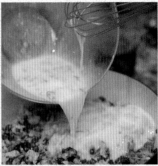

Add the egg mixture and mix to combine the ingredients before transferring to a baking dish.

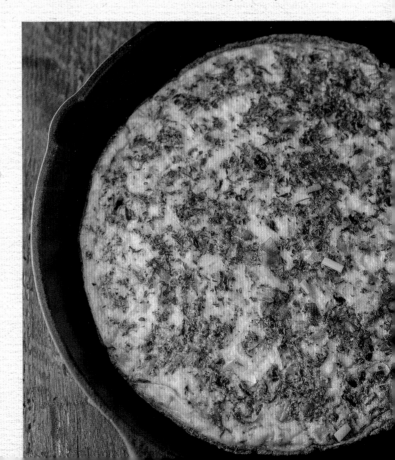

ZUCCHINI-BREAD FRENCH TOAST

I always double the zucchini bread recipe and make two loaves. We enjoy one immediately, and freeze the other—unless one of the kids claims it—so that when our family is home for the weekend or we have guests at our lake house I can just pull it out of the freezer and make French toast.

This is a truly gourmet breakfast or brunch. I recommend topping it with fresh fruit and a splash of pure maple syrup.

PALEO ZUCCHINI BREAD

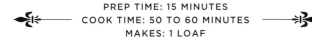

PREP TIME: 15 MINUTES
COOK TIME: 50 TO 60 MINUTES
MAKES: 1 LOAF

¾ cup (95 g) coconut flour
½ teaspoon sea salt
½ teaspoon baking powder
1 teaspoon baking soda
2 teaspoons cinnamon
1 teaspoon nutmeg
3 large eggs, room temperature
1 cup (250 ml) olive oil or melted coconut oil
½ cup (125 ml) honey
½ cup (125 ml) unsweetened applesauce
1 large zucchini, grated (about 1 cup or 150 g)
1 teaspoon good quality vanilla extract
¼ cup (25 g) walnuts (optional)

Preheat oven to 325°F (150°C)

Grease a loaf pan with melted coconut oil.

In a mixing bowl, sift together the coconut flour, salt, baking powder, baking soda, cinnamon and nutmeg.

Whisk eggs thoroughly in a separate bowl.

Fold the dry mixture into the eggs with a rubber spatula.

Mix in the oil, honey and applesauce, then add the zucchini and vanilla. Stir to combine. Add the walnuts, if using.

Pour the batter into the greased loaf pan and bake 55 to 60 minutes, or until a toothpick inserted into the middle comes out clean.

CINDY'S NOTE
You can make this French toast in advance. Just preheat the oven to 150°F (65°C) and place on a baking sheet until ready to serve. You can also sprinkle crushed nuts on the bread after dipping it in the eggs. My granddaughter likes her French toast with a little dark chocolate grated on top. Be creative!

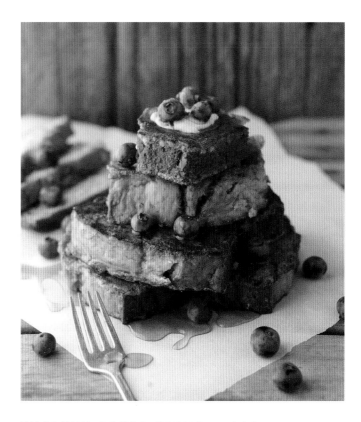

ZUCCHINI-BREAD FRENCH TOAST

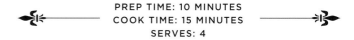

PREP TIME: 10 MINUTES
COOK TIME: 15 MINUTES
SERVES: 4

4 to 6 large eggs
Coconut oil, for frying
1 loaf zucchini bread (see recipe on this page), sliced
Cinnamon, for sprinkling
Unsalted butter, to taste
Pure maple syrup, to taste

Whisk the eggs in a large bowl.

Heat a large skillet over medium heat. Add a tablespoon or more of oil.

Dip the zucchini bread in beaten egg to coat both sides. Sprinkle both sides with cinnamon.

Place the dipped bread on the hot pan and cook each side for 2 to 3 minutes. Fry the bread in batches, adding more oil between each batch.

Top each piece of French toast with a little butter and serve with pure maple syrup.

EGGS BAKED IN TOMATOES ITALIAN-STYLE

This is especially nice to serve in the summer, when ripe tomatoes are available fresh from the garden or the farmers' market. It's one of those dishes that looks fancy, but isn't that difficult to make—perfect for brunch with friends!

When my husband is away on business I often make this for a simple dinner, sometimes adding salmon or leftovers from another meal.

 PREP TIME: 15 MINUTES
COOK TIME: 45 MINUTES
SERVES: 4

4 large ripe tomatoes
4 slices uncured bacon or pancetta
4 large eggs, at room temperature
2 green onions (scallions), green and white parts,
  chopped
1 clove garlic, minced
1 teaspoon sea salt, plus more for sprinkling
¾ teaspoon freshly ground black pepper
1 teaspoon dried basil
1 teaspoon dried parsley
¼ teaspoon dried red pepper flakes (optional)
1 tablespoon olive oil
Sriracha (optional for garnish)

Preheat the oven to 350°F (175°C).

Use a paring knife to cut the tops off the tomatoes, then scoop out the seeds and pulp with a spoon (refrigerate or freeze for future use in a sauce or soup). Set the tomato shells on a baking sheet lined with foil or parchment, or place them in individual ramekins.

Place a large skillet over medium heat. Add the bacon or pancetta slices and cook until crisp. Remove from the pan and let cool, then dice and set aside.

Whisk the eggs together in a mixing bowl. Add the green onions, garlic, salt, pepper, basil, parsley and red pepper flakes, if using. Stir in the diced bacon or pancetta.

Pour a little olive oil inside each of the tomato shells, and then lightly season each one with a pinch of salt.

Pour egg mixture into the tomato shells, dividing evenly between them. Bake for 35 to 40 minutes, or until eggs are fully cooked.

To serve, drizzle with a little olive oil and sriracha, if desired.

CINDY'S NOTE

If you are preparing this for Sunday brunch, you can whisk the eggs and other ingredients together the night before and store them in a sealed container. The tomato shells can also be prepared in advance; just season them lightly with salt and put them on a platter, cover with plastic wrap and refrigerate. In the morning, you can assemble them while the oven is preheating, then bake and serve.

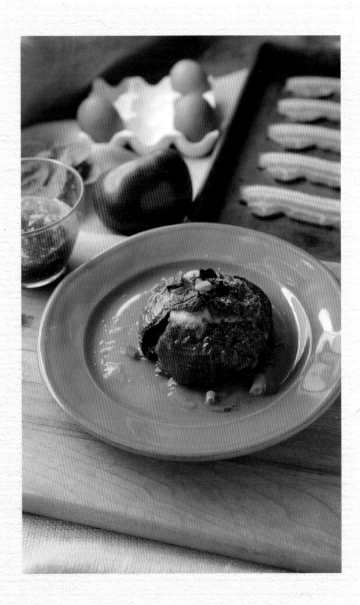

MUFFINS WITH PANCETTA & HERBS

*Some mornings we just want muffins and a cup of coffee.
Being Italian, I always have pancetta in my refrigerator.
Using fresh herbs in these muffins makes them extra special,
but if you don't have them handy, dried herbs are fine.*

 PREP TIME: 15 MINUTES
COOK TIME: 25 MINUTES
SERVES: 8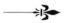

1 tablespoon coconut oil or ghee, plus more for the
  muffin tin
¼ lb (125 g) sliced pancetta, finely chopped
1 cup (100 g) almond flour
½ teaspoon baking soda
½ teaspoon sea salt
2 large eggs, at room temperature
½ teaspoon apple cider vinegar
1 tablespoon raw honey (preferably local)
1 tablespoon fresh thyme, chopped
1 tablespoon fresh parsley, chopped

Preheat oven to 350°F (175°C). Brush a muffin tin with
melted coconut oil.

Place a medium skillet over medium heat and add the
coconut oil or ghee. Once hot, add the chopped pancetta and
let cook until crisp, about 5 to 7 minutes. Remove from pan
and place on a paper-towel-lined plate to drain.

In a medium mixing bowl, combine the almond flour,
baking soda and salt.

In another medium mixing bowl, whisk together the eggs,
apple cider vinegar and honey. Add in the fresh herbs.

Fold the dry ingredients in the wet with a spatula until all
ingredients are incorporated. Stir in the pancetta.

Scoop equal amounts of batter into each muffin cup. Bake
for 15 minutes, or until brown around the edges.

Let cool for a few minutes, then enjoy.

CINDY'S NOTE

Pancetta is much easier to chop finely if you put
it in the freezer for 15 minutes first to firm it up.
And be sure to use a sharp chef's knife!

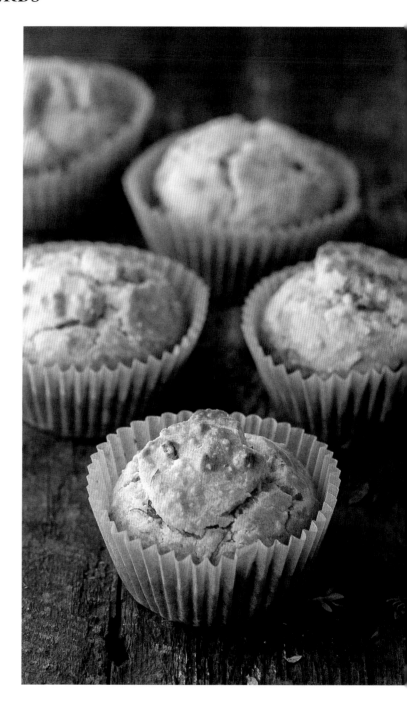

SUNBUTTER & MACADAMIA MUFFINS

Every afternoon around three o'clock I enjoy a cup of tea. I was rummaging around the pantry for something to make to go with it, and I came up with these muffins. Keeping a stocked pantry comes in handy when you want a healthy and satisfying muffin.

PREP TIME: 15 MINUTES
COOK TIME: 15 MINUTES
MAKES: 8 TO 10 MUFFINS

1 cup (100 g) almond flour
½ cup (500 g) coconut sugar
1 teaspoon baking soda
½ teaspoon baking powder
½ teaspoon sea salt
1 teaspoon cinnamon
3 large eggs, at room temperature
1 cup (250 g) sunflower-seed butter
⅓ cup (80 ml) melted coconut oil
½ teaspoon vanilla extract
¼ cup (50 g) macadamia nuts, crushed

Preheat oven to 350°F (175°C). Place 8 to 10 paper liners in the cups of an 8- or 12-cup muffin tin.

In a large mixing bowl, combine the almond flour, coconut sugar, baking soda, baking powder, sea salt and cinnamon.

Whisk the eggs together in a medium mixing bowl. Add the sunflower-seed butter, coconut oil and vanilla extract and whisk to blend.

Stir the egg mixture into the dry ingredients until thoroughly incorporated. Fold in the macadamia nuts.

Distribute the batter evenly in the muffin tin cups to make 8 to 10 muffins, depending on the size of the cups.

Bake for 15 to 18 minutes, or until a toothpick inserted in the center of a muffin comes out clean.

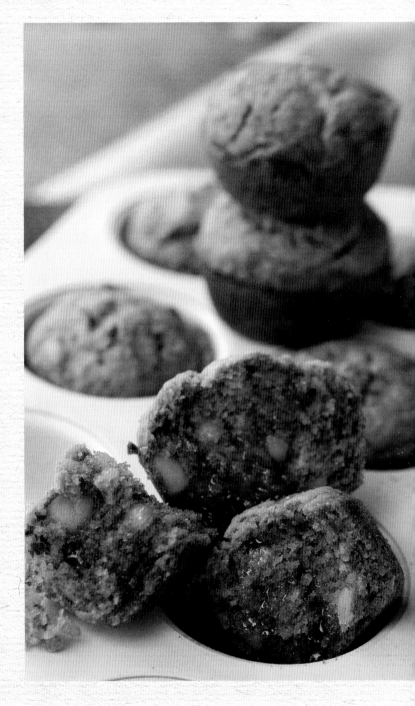

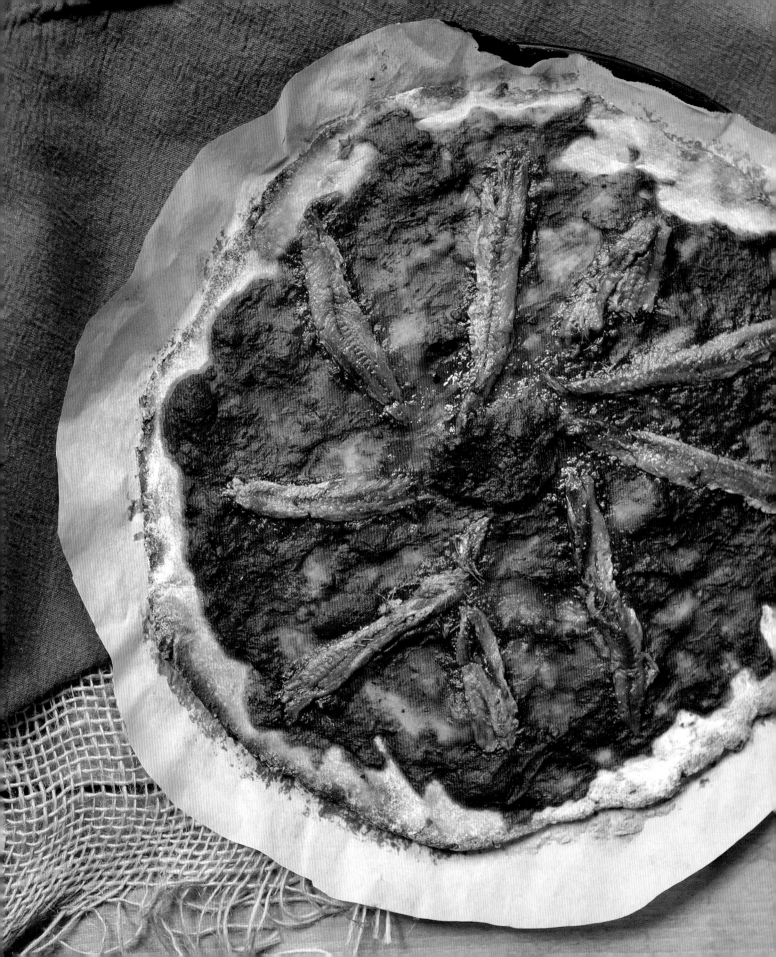

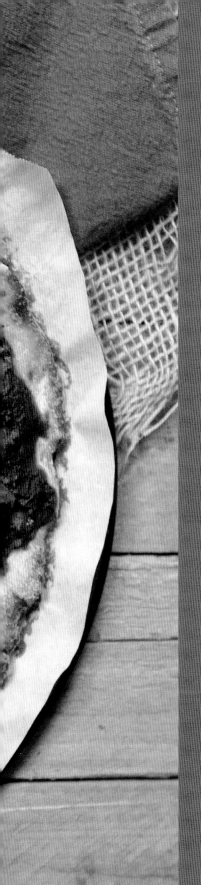

TUSCAN
FAVORITES

I added this section to share some of the
dishes that inspired me in Tuscany. These
recipes are all simple yet authentic—and,
of course, Paleo-friendly. The vibrant, fresh
flavors belie the simplicity of the preparations.
Get ready to impress your friends and family
and enjoy these recipes—preferably with a
glass of excellent Tuscan wine—and make
wonderful memories of your own!

STEAK TARTARE TOPPED WITH ARUGULA

It seems every restaurant in Tuscany has its own version of a steak tartare with arugula salad. Arugula, also known as rocket, is a nutritious green-leafy vegetable that's very popular in the Mediterranean. It has an assertive flavor that is outstanding in salads as well as cooked dishes. Young arugula leaves are especially tender and satisfying.

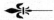 **PREP TIME: 15 MINUTES**
SERVES: 4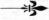

1 lb (500 g) beef tenderloin, trimmed
2 shallots, minced (about 3 tablespoons)
2 anchovy fillets, minced
1 tablespoon capers, small
1 teaspoon Dijon mustard
1 teaspoon sea salt
¾ teaspoon freshly ground black pepper
Juice of 1 lemon
½ cup (125 ml) extra-virgin olive oil
¼ lb (115 g) baby arugula (rocket)

Put the beef tenderloin through a meat grinder or slice it paper-thin. Set aside.

Combine the shallots, anchovies and capers in a medium wooden bowl. Mash against the sides of the bowl with a fork to make a paste.

In a small bowl, whisk the Dijon mustard, salt, pepper and lemon juice. Then, slowly add the olive oil while whisking continuously.

Add the beef to the dressing and mix gently to combine.

Arrange the arugula in a layer on a large serving platter. Top with the vinaigrette-dressed beef.

CINDY'S NOTE
If you don't have a meat grinder, try wrapping the beef and putting it in the freezer for about 15 minutes before slicing it. This makes it firmer, so it's easy to cut it into perfect thin slices.

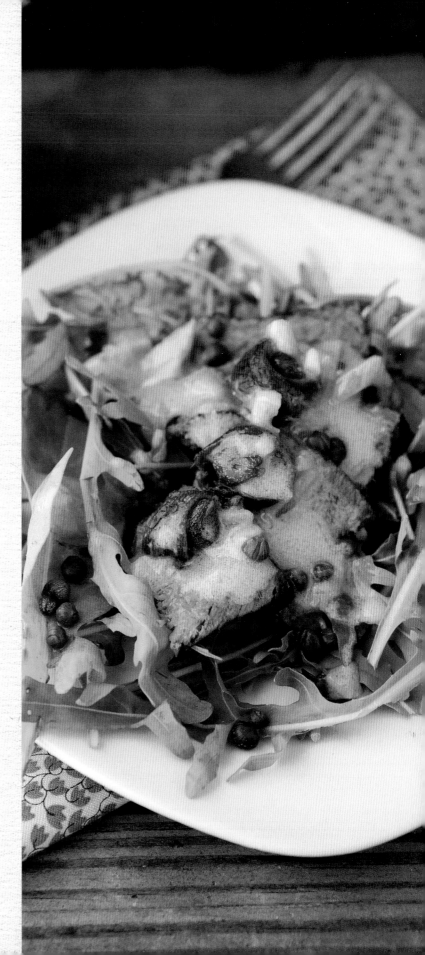

PAN-ROASTED GARLIC-SAGE QUAIL

Though it's not often served in the U.S., quail is very traditional in Italy. Be careful not to overcook the tiny birds, as they are delicate. This dish goes especially well with grilled eggplant, zucchini and red peppers.

 PREP TIME: 15 MINUTES
COOK TIME: 40 MINUTES
SERVES: 4

6 whole quails, rinsed and patted dry

2 teaspoons sea salt

1 teaspoon freshly ground black pepper

1 shallot, chopped (about 2 tablespoons)

8 fresh sage leaves

10 to 12 cloves garlic, peeled

¼ cup (60 ml) olive oil

Preheat oven to 350°F (175°C)

Place the quail in a 9 x 13-in (23 x 33-cm) baking dish.

Sprinkle the salt and pepper over the quail. Add the chopped shallot, sage leaves and whole garlic cloves.

Drizzle the olive oil over all.

Bake for 40 minutes. Serve with your favorite roasted vegetables.

CINDY'S TIP

Quail may be hard to find at your local grocery store. If you have trouble, try a specialty meat market, or check the freezer section of a larger upscale grocery store.

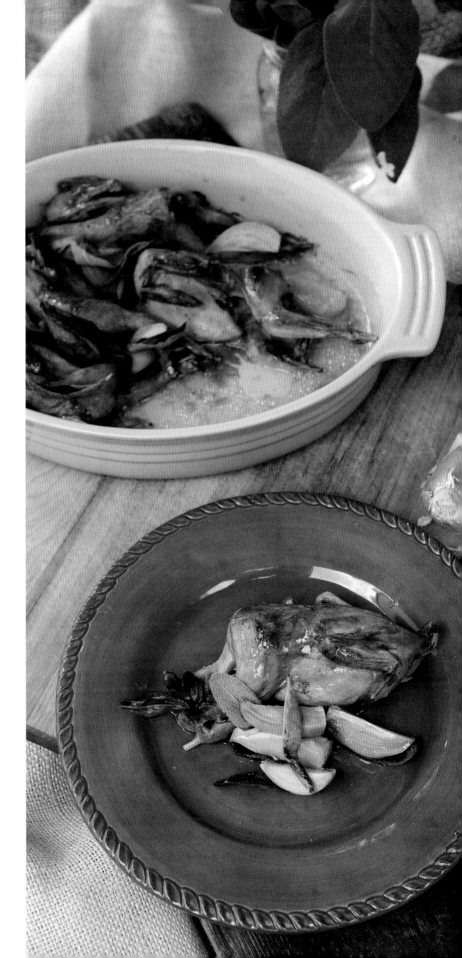

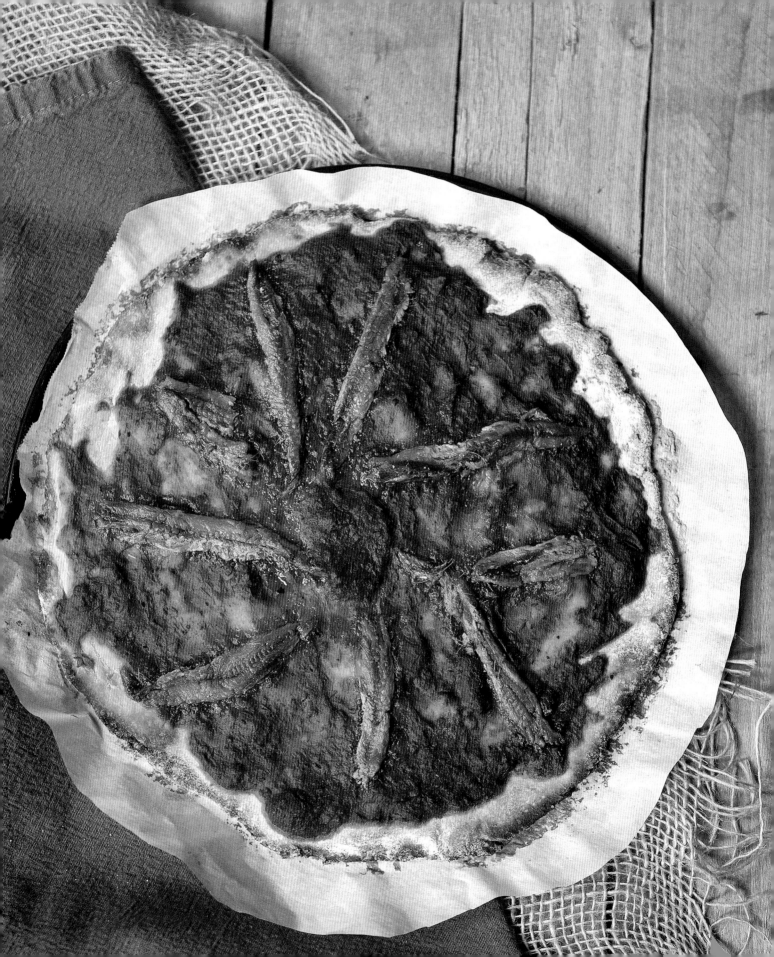

ANCHOVY PIZZA

My husband and I are creatures of habit. When we visit Tuscany, we order an anchovy pizza and a salad to share every day for lunch. Tuscan anchovy pizza is like no other: just a very thin crust with a delicate tomato sauce, and anchovies laid out beautifully on top. No cheese! I decided to develop a Paleo version that still evokes the original Tuscan flavor. Other toppings work too, but do give the anchovies a try.

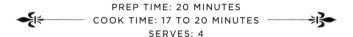

PREP TIME: 20 MINUTES
COOK TIME: 17 TO 20 MINUTES
SERVES: 4

2 teaspoons (1 package) active dry yeast

⅓ cup (80 ml) warm water

¾ cup (70 g) almond flour (plus extra for dusting)

¼ cup (30 g) coconut flour

⅔ cup (85 g) arrowroot flour

1 teaspoon sea salt, plus more for sprinkling

2 tablespoons coconut sugar

1 large egg, at room temperature

2½ teaspoons extra-virgin olive oil, plus more for drizzling

1 teaspoon apple cider vinegar

1 cup (250 ml) Five-Minute Pizza Sauce (see recipe on this page—or marinara sauce)

8 to 10 anchovies (from a can)

2 teaspoons dried oregano

Preheat oven to 450°F (230°C).

Combine the warm water and yeast in a glass measuring cup. Let sit for 10 minutes.

Sift the almond flour, coconut flour and salt together in a medium mixing bowl. Add the coconut sugar and mix with a fork to remove any lumps.

Whisk the egg into the flour mixture, then add the oil and apple cider vinegar.

Add the yeast mixture and stir with a spatula or wooden spoon, then knead by hand for 7 to 10 minutes.

Line a baking sheet with parchment paper. Dust the parchment with a little almond flour, then place the dough in the center. Wet your hands with cold water and flatten the dough, pressing it outward, to create a round crust.

Bake for 7 minutes. Remove the crust from the oven and flip it over.

Spread the pizza sauce or marinara over the crust, then arrange the anchovies on top. Sprinkle with oregano and a little sea salt. Return to the oven and bake for another 8 to 10 minutes.

Drizzle the pizza with extra-virgin olive oil before serving. Enjoy with a glass of Montepulciano.

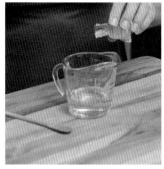

Add the yeast to the warm water.

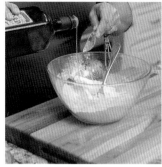

Combine the flours in a separate bowl. Add the egg to the flour, then add the oil and vinegar to the flour mixture.

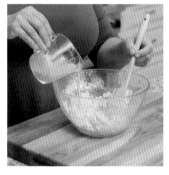

Mix to combine the ingredients. Pour in the yeast mixture and stir to incorporate.

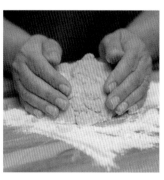

Knead the resulting dough.

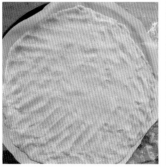

Form the dough into a round crust.

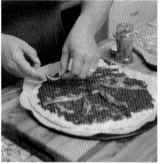

After baking and flipping the dough, spread the pizza sauce on top. Lay the anchovies over the sauce and put the pizza back in the oven.

FIVE-MINUTE PIZZA SAUCE

In a medium saucepan, combine ½ cup (120 g) crushed tomatoes, 1 tablespoon tomato paste, ½ teaspoon chopped garlic, ¾ teaspoon sea salt and ½ teaspoon each of oregano, basil and parsley. Bring to a boil, then simmer until ready to use. Save leftover sauce for dipping.

ROMAN BRAISED EGGPLANT

Eggplant is one of my favorite vegetables, and I have a number of ways of preparing it. I always turn to this one when I need an easy side dish using eggplant and other ingredients that I always have on hand.

 PREP TIME: 15 MINUTES
COOK TIME: 1 HOUR
SERVES: 4

2 medium eggplants, sliced in half lengthwise

½ cup (125 ml) olive oil, divided

2 teaspoons sea salt, divided

¾ teaspoon freshly ground pepper, plus more

1 yellow onion, roughly chopped

1 red bell pepper, sliced

4 thin slices prosciutto, chopped

2 cloves garlic, minced

One 15-oz (425-g) can petite diced tomatoes, drained

1½ teaspoons dried parsley

1 teaspoon dried basil

1 teaspoon dried thyme

¼ teaspoon dried red pepper flakes (optional)

2 tablespoons capers

Preheat oven to 350°F (175°C).

Spread 2 tablespoons of the olive oil on the bottom of a large baking dish.

Scoop out the flesh from each eggplant half with a spoon, leaving a ½-in (1.25-cm) layer. Set the flesh aside. Place the eggplants on the baking dish face-up.

Season the surface of the eggplant with half the salt and pepper, then drizzle about 2 tablespoons of the olive oil over.

Chop up the eggplant flesh and place in a medium mixing bowl.

Add the onion, bell pepper, prosciutto, garlic, tomatoes, parsley, basil, thyme, red pepper flakes and capers. Combine well.

Scoop an equal amount of the tomato mixture into each eggplant and top with the remaining salt and pepper.

Drizzle the remaining ¼ cup olive oil over the eggplants and bake for 45 to 55 minutes.

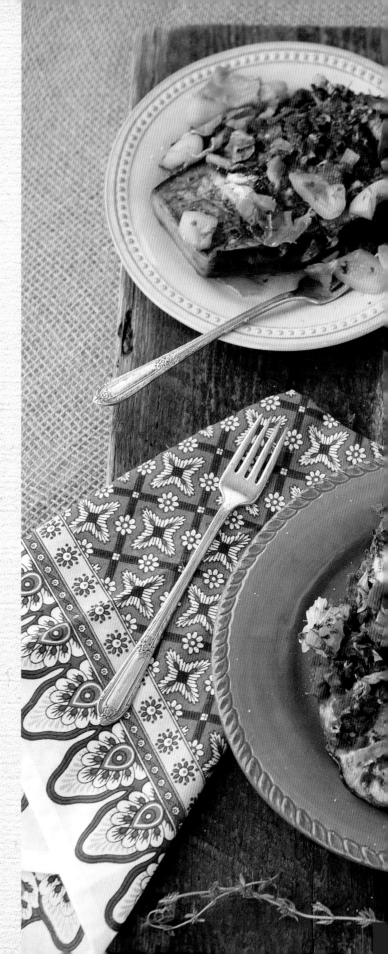

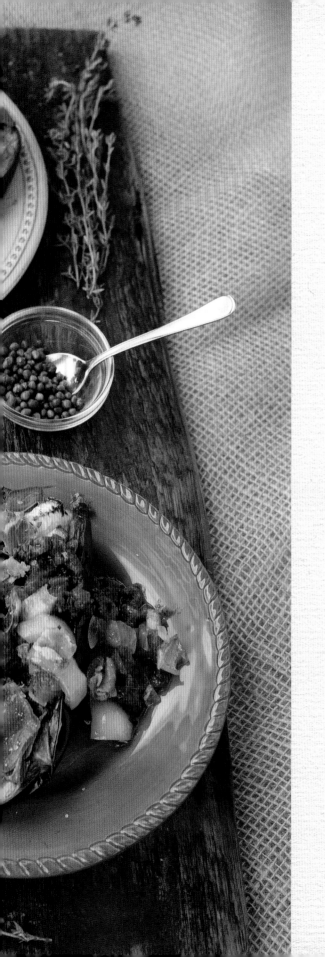

FLANK STEAK WITH SALSA VERDE

There are many ways to prepare flank steak. It cooks so fast you can have dinner ready in no time at all. I like to put it in a resealable plastic bag with salt, pepper, garlic powder and olive oil and let it marinate all day in the refrigerator. All you have to do is heat the grill and prepare the Salsa Verde, and this quick dish can be on the table in a jiffy!

 PREP TIME: 20 MINUTES
COOK TIME: 20 MINUTES
SERVES: 4

1 flank steak (about 1½ lbs / 680 g), trimmed
2 tablespoons plus ½ cup (50 ml) extra-virgin olive oil
1½ teaspoons sea salt, divided
1¼ teaspoons freshly ground black pepper, divided
1 teaspoon garlic powder
1 small onion, coarsely chopped
1 clove garlic, peeled and chopped
2 tablespoons capers, drained
¾ cup (15 g) chopped fresh parsley
2 teaspoons fresh lemon juice
¼ teaspoon dried red pepper flakes
1 tinned anchovy fillet, rinsed, dried and finely chopped, (optional)

Lay the steak on a board or large platter. Sprinkle both sides with the 2 tablespoons extra-virgin olive oil, then season with 1 teaspoon of the salt, ¼ teaspoon of the pepper and the garlic powder. Set aside.

Preheat a gas grill to medium-high heat.

Combine the onion, garlic cloves, capers, parsley, lemon juice, red pepper flakes and anchovy fillet in a food processor and pulse 3 times. Continue pulsing while slowly adding in the remaining ½ cup of extra-virgin olive oil. Add the remaining ½ teaspoons of sea salt and pepper and pulse 2 more times. Taste and adjust seasonings if necessary.

Transfer the Salsa Verde to a bowl and set aside.

Grill the steak for 4 to 6 minutes per side (for medium-rare).

Let stand for 5 to 7 minutes on a wooden board, then thinly slice the cooked steak against the grain. Serve on a large platter with the Salsa Verde (page 32) alongside.

CINDY'S NOTE
Don't shy away from the anchovy fillet—it makes this Salsa Verde extra special. It doesn't add a fishy taste, but really deepens the flavor of the sauce. If you don't have anchovies handy, you can use ½ teaspoon of anchovy paste.

RIBOLLITA

Ribollita is a thick Tuscan stew filled with dark green beans and vegetables. It's prepared by bringing the ingredients to a boil, letting them cool down, and then cooking them again. This is my Paleo version of the traditional stew. I generally use a combination of cabbage, kale and Swiss chard, but any other dark leafy greens such as chicory can be used as well.

PREP TIME: 20 MINUTES
COOK TIME: 40 MINUTES
REST TIME: OVERNIGHT
SERVES: 6

3 tablespoons olive oil

1 large yellow onion, diced

2 carrots, peeled and sliced

2 large stalks celery, chopped

1 large white sweet potato, chopped

2 cups (200 g) cabbage, coarsely chopped

5 leaves kale, trimmed and chopped

4 leaves Swiss chard, trimmed and chopped

4 cloves garlic, minced

1 teaspoon sea salt, plus more

1 teaspoon freshly ground black pepper, plus more

8 cups (2 liters) low sodium chicken broth

One 28-oz (800-g) can petite diced tomatoes

3 fresh sage leaves

3 bay leaves

1 teaspoon sea salt

¾ teaspoon freshly ground black pepper

Extra-virgin olive oil, for drizzling

Place a large cast-iron pan or soup pot over medium-high heat. Add the olive oil. Once hot, add the onions and cook for about 5 minutes, until translucent.

Add the carrots, celery and sweet potato. Continue cooking for 5 minutes more.

Add the cabbage, kale, Swiss chard and garlic. Stir well with a wooden spoon. Cover and continue cooking for 10 minutes.

Pour in the chicken broth and the diced tomatoes. Add the sage and bay leaves and stir.

Season with salt and pepper.

Bring to a boil, then cover and reduce heat to low. Simmer for 20 minutes. Remove from heat and let cool.

Refrigerate overnight. Before serving, place over medium heat for 20 minutes or until hot.

To serve, ladle the Ribollita into bowls and drizzle extra-virgin olive oil on top.

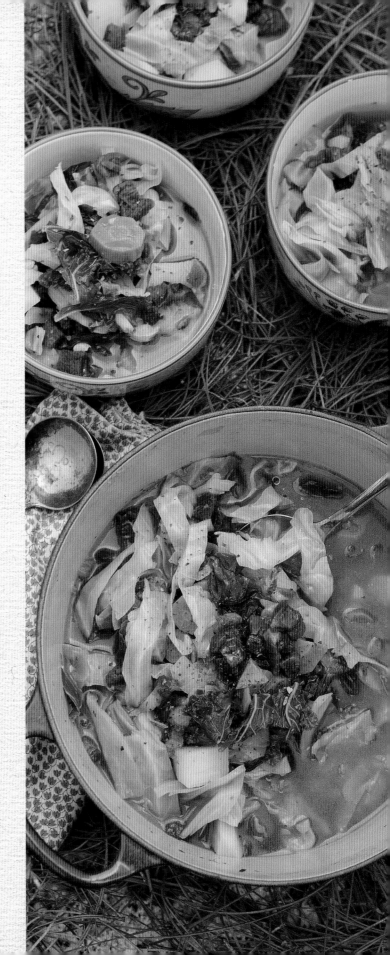

ITALIAN HERO SANDWICH ROLLS

Nana used to make a large Italian sandwich for lunch on the weekend. She called it an "airplane" for some reason— maybe because it was big enough to serve an airplane full of passengers. An individual-serving sized sandwich like this is called a "hero." I devised this recipe when I wanted to make a Paleo sandwich bread to use for heroes, and I'm extremely happy with the result.

PREP TIME: 15 MINUTES
COOK TIME: 25 MINUTES
SERVES: 4 ROLLS

1 cup (140 g) raw cashews

⅓ cup (40 g) coconut flour

¼ cup (30 g) almond flour

1 teaspoon sea salt

1 teaspoon baking soda

3 large eggs, at room temperature

¾ teaspoon apple cider vinegar

¼ cup (65 ml) full-fat coconut milk

5 tablespoons unsalted butter, melted and cooled (divided)

1 teaspoon dried basil

1 teaspoon dried parsley

Preheat oven to 325°F (160°C).

Line a baking sheet with parchment paper.

Place the cashews in a food processor and process until very smooth.

In the bowl of a stand mixer or a medium mixing bowl, combine the pulverized cashews, coconut flour, almond flour, salt and baking soda. If using a mixer, turn it on low.

Keeping the mixer on low or stirring with a wooden spoon, add one egg at a time, then add the apple cider vinegar, coconut milk and 4 tablespoons of the melted butter. The ingredients will form a stiff dough.

Remove the dough from the mixer or bowl and divide into 4 balls.

Form each ball into a longish roll, then place on the parchment paper and finish shaping into a little sandwich roll.

Brush the rolls with the remaining 1 tablespoon melted butter, then sprinkle with basil and parsley. You can also add a little extra sea salt.

Bake for 25 minutes. Allow to cool before slicing lengthwise to make Italian hero sandwiches.

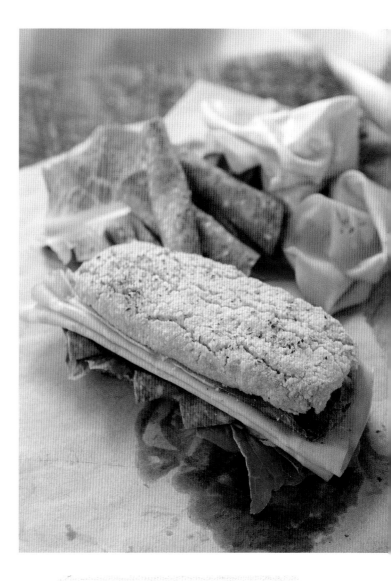

MAKE THE PERFECT ITALIAN SANDWICH

Layer Genoa salami, mortadella and hot or sweet capicola from your local Italian market onto a hero sandwich roll. Top with lettuce, tomato, thinly sliced red onion and dried oregano, then drizzle with extra-virgin olive oil or spread on Paleo Mayonnaise (page 32). I usually add pickles and olives, too.

CINDY'S NOTE

These rolls should be used soon after they are made, as they harden over time. When this happened to me, I put it the stale roll in the food processor and turned it into bread crumbs for my chicken Parmesan!

COD FLORENTINE

This recipe is not only delicious, but also beautiful to look at. Italians do eat with their eyes; if it looks good, we know it will taste good too. You can use cod, haddock, flounder or any other white flaky fish for this recipe. The combination of spinach, garlic and herbs makes it a standout dish.

 PREP TIME: 15 MINUTES
COOK TIME: 10 MINUTES
SERVES: 4

Four 7-oz (200-g) cod fillets (28 oz / 800 g total)
1 teaspoon sea salt, divided
¾ teaspoon freshly ground black pepper, divided
2 tablespoons coconut oil, unsalted butter or olive oil
2 tablespoons fresh lemon juice
1 lemon, sliced
5 cups (175 g) baby spinach
3 cloves garlic, minced
1 teaspoon dried basil
1 teaspoon dried parsley
½ teaspoon dried red pepper flakes (optional)
Extra-virgin olive oil, for drizzling

Preheat oven to 325°F (160°F).

Place the cod fillets on a platter. Season both sides with ½ teaspoon of the salt and ½ teaspoon of the black pepper.

Place a large oven-safe skillet over medium heat. Add the oil or butter. When hot, add the cod. Cook for about 3 minutes, then turn over. Sprinkle with the lemon juice and add the lemon slices to the pan. Remove the cod from the pan and tent with foil.

In a large bowl, combine the spinach, garlic, basil, parsley, red pepper flakes, remaining ½ teaspoon of the sea salt and remaining ½ teaspoon of the freshly ground pepper.

Cover the cod with the spinach mixture. Place in the oven and bake for 7 to 10 minutes.

Before serving, drizzle a little extra-virgin olive oil over the fish.

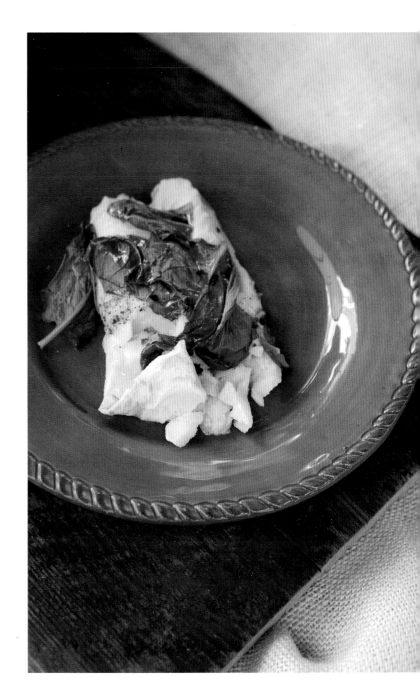

CREAMY SRIRACHA SHRIMP COCKTAIL

This is a quick and easy appetizer. If you keep frozen cooked shrimp in your freezer, you can thaw the shrimp the night before. If you need them sooner, just set the bag in a bowl of cold water to quick-thaw the shrimp.

 PREP TIME: 10 MINUTES
SERVES: 6

½ cup (100 g) Paleo Mayonnaise (page 32)
Juice of 1 lime (about 1 tablespoon)
2 tablespoons sriracha hot sauce
½ teaspoon sea salt
2 green onions (scallions), finely chopped
  (reserve a few for garnish if desired)
1 lb (500 g) cooked shrimp, fresh or frozen

In a small bowl, combine the mayonnaise, lime juice, sriracha, sea salt and green onions.

Arrange shrimp on a platter or in a glass, then place the creamy sriracha at the center.

To make this appetizer extra special, add a few extra drops of sriracha and scatter green onions over the shrimp before serving.

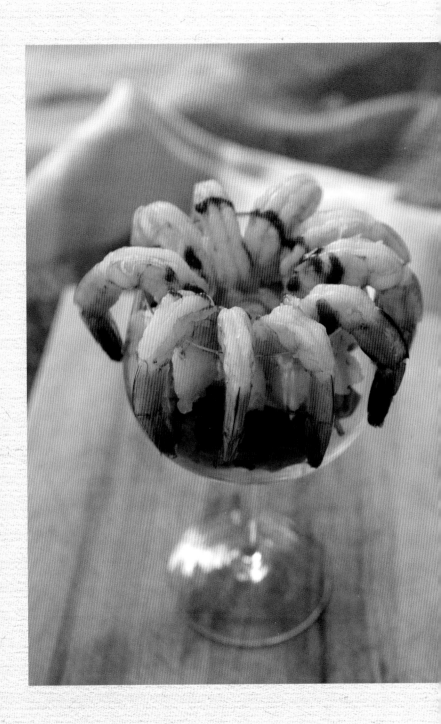

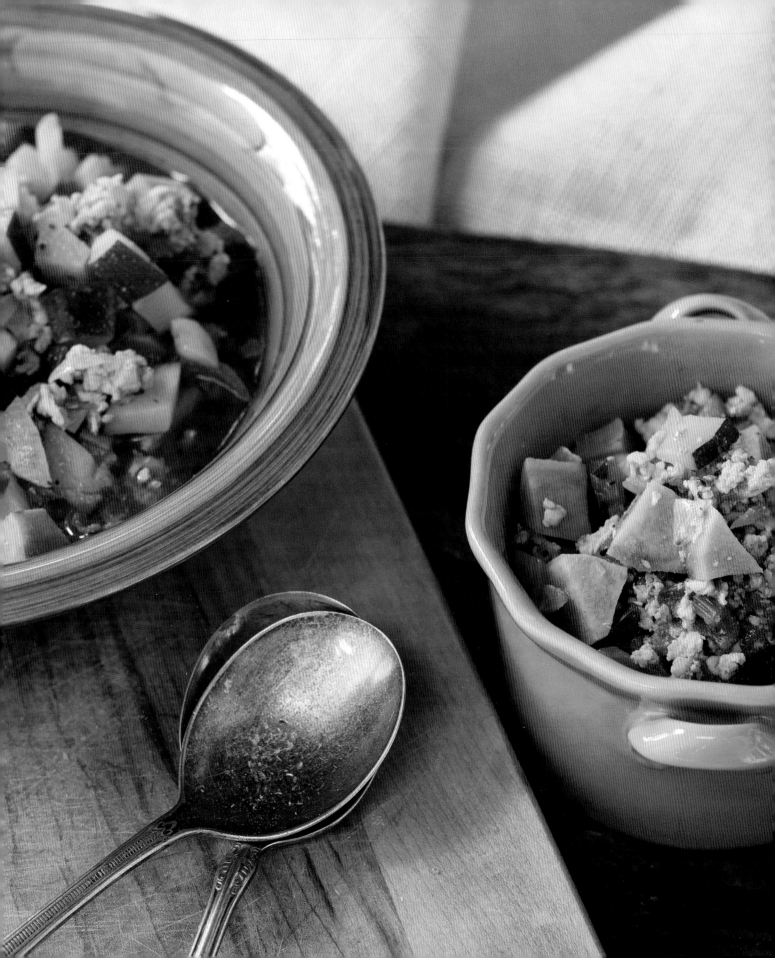

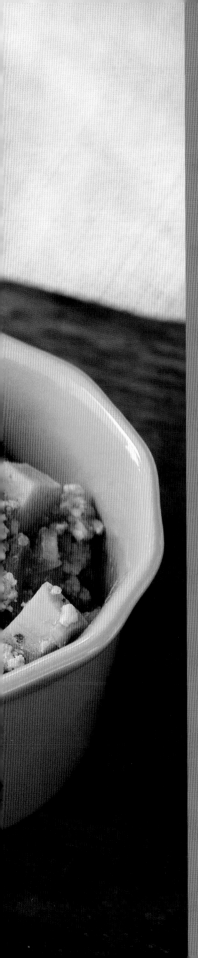

SOUPS, STEWS & CHILI

On the weekends, Nana would always ask if we
wanted soup for lunch. Even as an adult,
I sometimes just eat a bowl of soup at midday,
and it's plenty for me. It's about how many
courses you eat in a day; smaller, more frequent
servings can be satisfying.

I prepare soups, stews and chili in a slow
cooker or in a large pot that sits simmering on
the stove all day. The aromas waft through the
house, drawing people to the kitchen. Sitting down
in the midst of a busy day to enjoy a small cup
from the pot can be a great refresher.

Most soups, stews and chili taste even better
the next day, since the flavors continue to marry
and improve overnight. You can also store
portions in the freezer for a quick meal when
you don't feel like cooking.

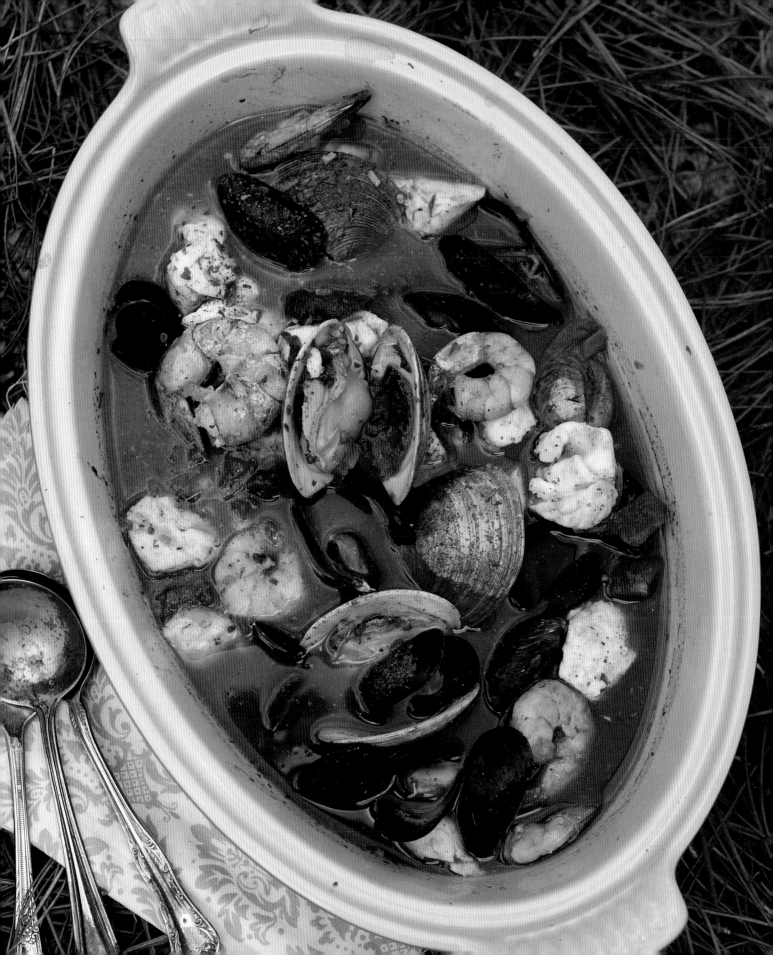

TUSCAN FISH SOUP

Though I call it a soup, this is more like a stew. We often had this on Sundays and holidays when I was growing up. You can use different kinds of fish in this soup to make it your own. Try topping it with capers before serving!

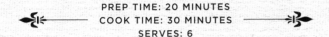

PREP TIME: 20 MINUTES
COOK TIME: 30 MINUTES
SERVES: 6

5 tablespoons olive oil

1 medium yellow onion, chopped

4 cloves garlic, minced

1 lb (500 g) mussels, scrubbed, and debearded

1 lb (500 g) clams, scrubbed

1 cup (250 ml) dry white wine

1 cup (225 g) Italian peeled tomatoes, drained and chopped

¼ cup (5 g) flat-leaf parsley, finely chopped

12 oz (350 g) halibut, cut into 2-in (5-cm) pieces

8 oz (250 g) large shrimp, peeled and deveined

1½ teaspoons sea salt

¾ teaspoon freshly ground black pepper

1 cup (250 ml) low sodium chicken or vegetable broth

Place a large cast-iron pot or soup pot over medium heat. When hot, add the olive oil.

Add in onion and cook for about 3 minutes. Add the garlic and cook for an additional 30 seconds.

Increase the heat to high, then add the mussels, clams and wine and cook, stirring frequently, until the shells begin to open.

Continue cooking until the liquid is reduced by half, then add the tomatoes and parsley. Cover and bring to a boil.

Reduce the heat to medium and add the halibut, shrimp, salt and pepper; return to a boil. Add the chicken or vegetable broth and simmer until the fish is cooked, about 7 minutes.

Bring the pot to the center of the table and let everyone serve themselves with a slotted spoon. Have a ladle handy so people can take as much broth as they want.

CINDY'S NOTE

As mentioned above, I like to add capers before serving. I also put a bottle of extra-virgin olive oil next to the pot to drizzle on top of the soup.

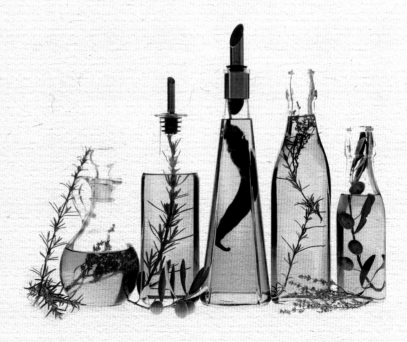

ZUCCHINI LEEK SOUP

This recipe was an experiment with zucchini and leeks that I had handy in the house. I was extremely impressed with the wonderful flavors created. I hope you enjoy this soup as much as we do in our house.

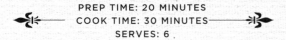

PREP TIME: 20 MINUTES
COOK TIME: 30 MINUTES
SERVES: 6

3 tablespoons olive oil

2 large leeks, rinsed and thinly sliced

2 large zucchinis, diced

5 cloves garlic, minced

2½ cups (625 ml) low-sodium chicken broth

3 tablespoons fresh parsley, chopped

1 teaspoon sea salt

¾ teaspoon freshly ground black pepper

2 tablespoons extra-virgin olive oil

Place a large cast-iron pot over medium heat. Add the olive oil. Once hot, add the leeks and cook, stirring often with a wooden spoon, for about 5 minutes, or until they begin to brown.

Add the zucchini and garlic. Continue cooking for another 5 minutes or until the zucchini is tender.

Add the chicken broth, parsley, salt and pepper. Bring to a boil, then remove from heat.

Puree the soup with an immersion blender, or transfer to a blender, puree, and return to the pot. Reduce the heat to low.

Taste and adjust seasonings as necessary. Ladle into bowls and drizzle extra-virgin olive oil over the top to serve.

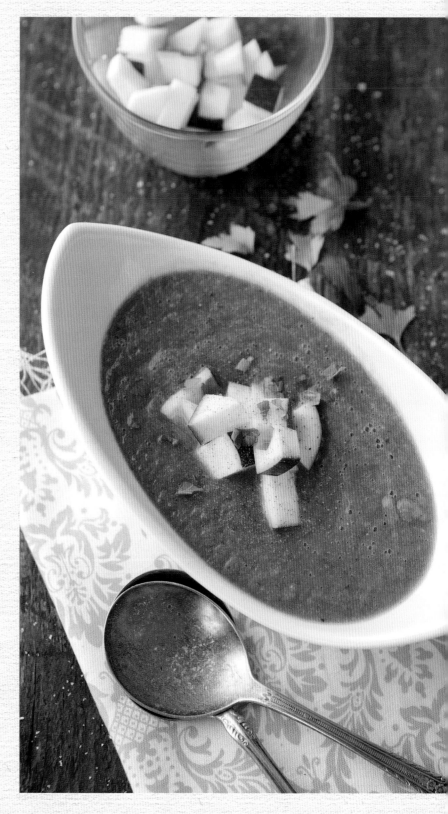

MINESTRONE

This classic Italian soup is a wonderful antidote for cold weather. It's hearty and full of flavor, so it's perfect for a family dinner. I add chopped kale to make it even more substantial.

PREP TIME: 20 MINUTES
COOK TIME: 30 MINUTES
SERVES: 6

2 tablespoons olive oil

1 large yellow onion, diced

3 cloves garlic, minced

2 stalks celery, diced

1 large carrot, diced

1 cup (150 g) fresh green beans, trimmed and cut into ½-in (1.25-cm) lengths

1 teaspoon dried basil

1 teaspoon dried oregano

½ teaspoon dried red pepper flakes (optional)

1½ teaspoons sea salt

1 teaspoon freshly ground black pepper

One 28-oz ounce (800-kg) can petite diced tomatoes

One 14-oz (400-ml) ounce can crushed tomatoes

7 cups (1.65 liters) low-sodium chicken broth

2 cups (100 g) kale, rib removed and chopped

Place a large cast-iron pot or soup pot over medium heat. Once hot, add the olive oil.

Add the onion and cook until translucent, about 3 minutes. Add the garlic and cook for 30 seconds.

Add the celery and carrots and continue cooking for about 5 minutes, stirring often with a wooden spoon.

Stir in the green beans, basil, oregano, red pepper flakes (if using), salt and pepper. Let cook for 3 minutes.

Add the diced tomatoes, crushed tomatoes and chicken broth to the pot. Bring to a boil, then add the kale.

Reduce the heat to low and allow to simmer, covered, for 10 minutes.

Taste and adjust seasonings if necessary.

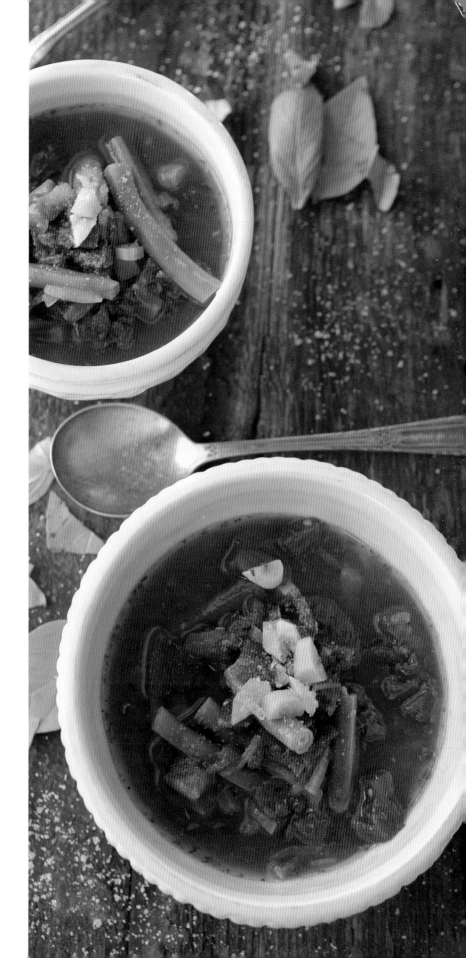

TUSCAN STEW WITH SAUSAGE & KALE

This stew is filling and delicious. I often make it on weekends, and just keep it simmering on the stove all day. I leave out bowls and a ladle so anyone can scoop some out and enjoy it whenever they want.

 PREP TIME: 20 MINUTES
COOK TIME: 40 MINUTES
SERVES: 6

2 to 3 tablespoons olive oil

1 lb (500 g) pork or chicken sausage, casings removed

1 large onion, finely chopped

1 teaspoon sea salt

¾ teaspoon freshly ground black pepper

2 cloves garlic, chopped

2 stalks celery, diced

1 carrot, peeled and diced

2 tablespoons tomato paste

One 15-oz (425-g) can petite diced tomatoes

5 cups (1.25 liters) chicken or vegetable stock

1 teaspoon dried basil

1 teaspoon dried thyme

1 bunch kale, ribs removed, chopped

Heat a large Dutch oven or pot over medium-high heat.

Add the olive oil. When hot, add the sausage and cook for 7 or 8 minutes. Use a wooden spoon to break up the sausage as it cooks.

Add the onion, salt, pepper, garlic, celery and carrot and cook, stirring, for about 3 minutes. Lower the heat to medium.

Add the tomato paste a spoonful at a time, pressing it against the sides of the pot as you stir to eliminate lumps.

Stir in the diced tomatoes, chicken broth, basil and thyme. Cover and let cook for about 10 minutes.

Toss in the kale and continue cooking for another 10 minutes.

Serve immediately or keep at a low simmer until ready to ladle into bowls.

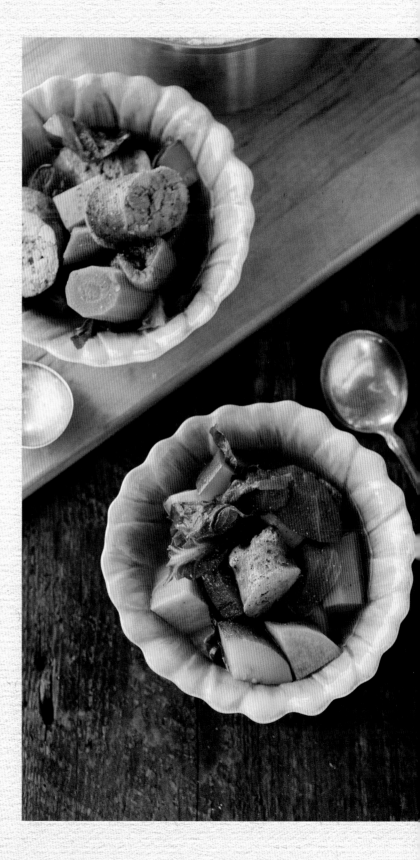

TUSCAN CHICKEN & VEGETABLE CHILI

Using ground chicken made from dark meat brings such great flavor to this chili. There's truly nothing better than a pot of chili simmering on the stove on a Sunday!

 PREP TIME: 10 MINUTES
COOK TIME: 30 MINUTES
SERVES: 6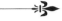

1½ tablespoons olive oil

1 lb (500 g) ground chicken (from dark meat, if possible)

1 teaspoon sea salt

¾ teaspoon freshly ground black pepper

1 small yellow onion, diced

2 small carrots, diced

2 stalks celery, diced

1 small zucchini, diced

2 cloves garlic, minced

1 teaspoon dried thyme

1 teaspoon dried parsley

½ teaspoon dried sage

3 cups (750 ml) low-sodium chicken broth or vegetable broth

One 15-oz (450-g) can petite diced tomatoes

2 cups (60 g) baby spinach leaves

2 cups (200 g) thinly sliced cabbage

Place a large Dutch oven or soup pot over medium-high heat. Add the olive oil.

When the oil is hot, add the ground chicken, salt and pepper and cook for about 5 minutes. Use a wooden spoon to break up the chicken as it cooks.

Stir in the onion, carrots, celery, zucchini, garlic, thyme, parsley and sage. Cook for another 5 minutes.

Pour in the broth and add the diced tomatoes, including the juice. Stir to combine, then cover and bring to a boil.

Add the spinach and cabbage, then cover and continue cooking for 10 minutes.

Serve or keep simmering over low heat until ready to enjoy!

CINDY'S NOTE

If you want to prepare dinner well ahead of time, this is a great recipe to make in a slow-cooker. First, brown the chicken in a skillet, then put it in the slow-cooker along with all other ingredients except the spinach and cabbage.

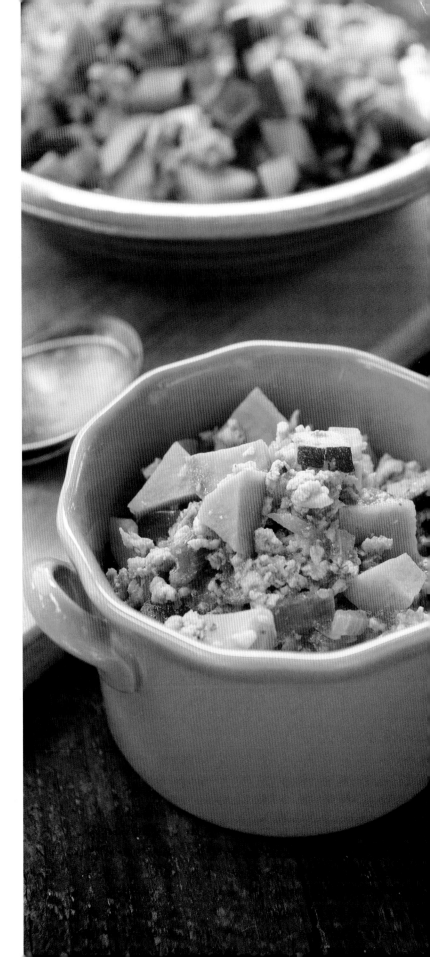

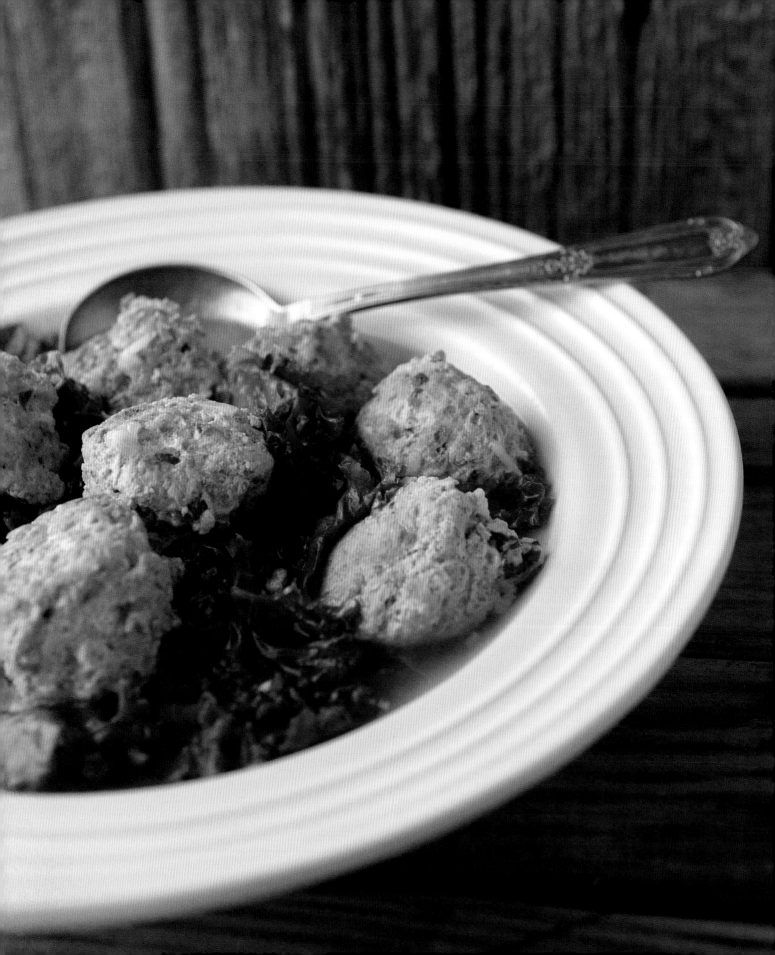

MEATBALL & KALE SOUP

I find that using ground turkey in this soup gives it a lighter flavor—but it's still a wonderfully satisfying dish.

PREP TIME: 20 MINUTES
COOK TIME: 30 MINUTES
SERVES: 6

1 lb (500 g) ground turkey

2 tablespoons chopped fresh flat-leaf parsley

2 tablespoons dried basil

1½ teaspoons sea salt, divided

1 teaspoon freshly ground black pepper, divided

5 cloves garlic, minced and divided

1 large egg

4 tablespoons olive oil, divided

½ cup (80 g) shallots, chopped

4 cups (250 g) kale, trimmed and chopped

¼ teaspoon dried red pepper flakes

5 cups (1.25 liters) low-sodium chicken broth

In a large bowl, combine the ground turkey, parsley, basil, 1 teaspoon of the sea salt, ½ teaspoon of the pepper, a bit more than half of the garlic and the egg. Combine gently, at first mixing with a fork then using your hands. Do not overmix.

Scoop out about 2 tablespoons of the turkey mixture and roll into a ball. Repeat to make about 20 meatballs.

Heat a large pot over medium-high heat. Add 2 tablespoons of the olive oil; when hot, add meatballs in batches and cook until brown, about 7 minutes. Add more oil between batches.

Set the cooked meatballs on a plate until you finish the last batch, then return all the meatballs to the pot.

Add the shallots and remaining garlic to the pot and stir gently, being careful not to break the meatballs.

Add the kale, red pepper flakes and chicken stock.

Reduce heat to medium-low and cover. Allow to cook for 20 minutes. Taste and adjust seasonings, if necessary, before serving.

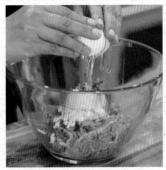

Put the ground turkey in the bowl and then add the parsley, basil, freshly ground black pepper, chopped garlic and an egg. Mix to combine the ingredients.

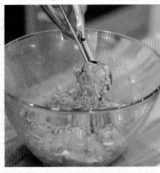

Combine the flours in a separate bowl Add the egg to the flour add the oil to the flour mixture.

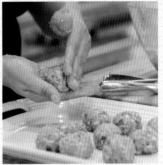

Form the meatballs.

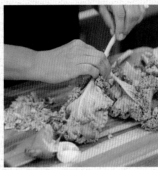

Chop the shallots and the kale.

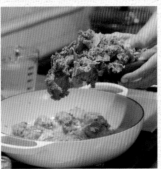

Add the oil to a pan over medium heat. Cook the meatballs in batches. Return all the meatballs to the pan and add the shallots and garlic. Add the kale.

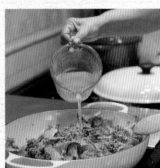

Add the broth, then stir and cover. Simmer until done.

TUSCAN TOMATO SOUP

This classic rustic Tuscan tomato soup is called pappa al pomodoro *in Italy. Scattering diced avocados on top makes it even better.*

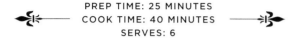

PREP TIME: 25 MINUTES
COOK TIME: 40 MINUTES
SERVES: 6

3 tablespoons olive oil
1 large yellow onion, shredded
1 carrot, peeled and shredded
3 cloves garlic, minced
1 teaspoon sea salt
½ teaspoon freshly ground black pepper
One 28-oz (800-g) can crushed tomatoes (try to get an imported Italian brand such as San Marzano)
2 cups (500 ml) chicken stock.
¼ cup (65 ml) Italian red wine
1 ripe avocado
Juice of 1 lime
1-2 tablespoons extra-virgin olive oil

Place a large cast-iron pan or soup pot over medium-high heat. Once the pan is hot, add the olive oil and let it heat for about 10 seconds. Add the onion and carrots. Cook for about 1 minute, then add the minced garlic, salt and pepper and cook for another 30 seconds.

Add the tomatoes, chicken stock and red wine. Bring to a boil, then reduce heat to low. Cover and simmer for 30 minutes.

While the soup is simmering, halve the avocado and remove the pit. With a sharp knife, crosshatch the avocado flesh down to the skin, then use a large spoon to scoop out the resulting cubed avocado into a bowl. Squeeze the lime juice over and mix gently.

Ladle the soup into bowls. Top with avocado and drizzle a little extra-virgin olive oil over to serve.

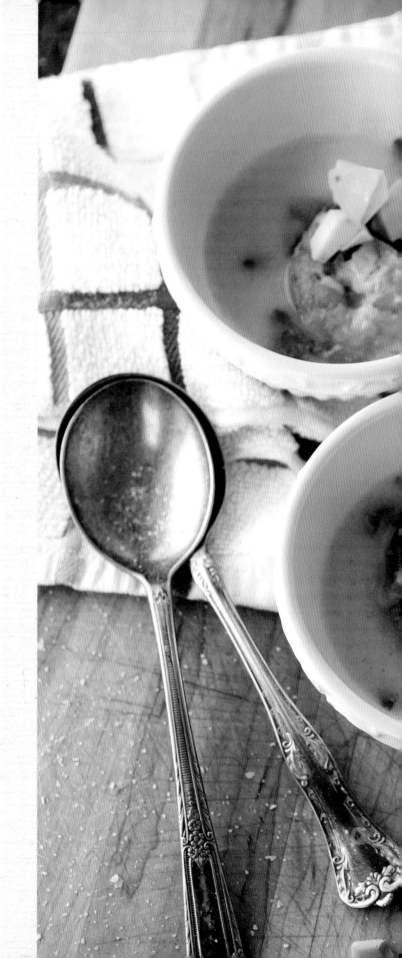

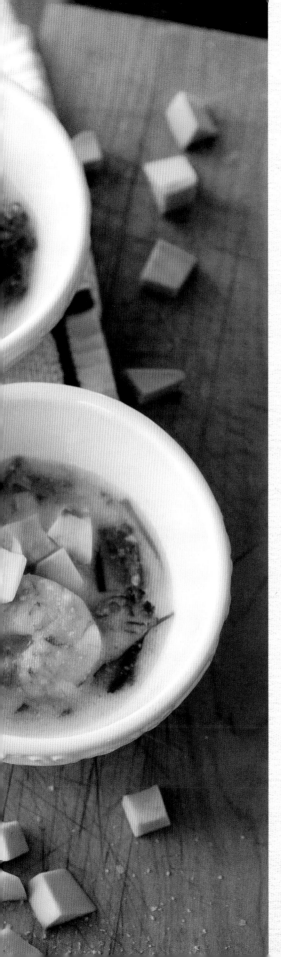

LEMON, SPINACH & PRAWN SOUP

The secret to making this creamy soup is to put a can of coconut milk in the refrigerator the night before. When you open the can, the cream will be on top. Scoop it out and save the watery liquid for another recipe.

 PREP TIME: 20 MINUTES
COOK TIME: 25 MINUTES
SERVES: 6

3 tablespoons olive or coconut oil, divided
1 tablespoon unsalted butter or ghee
1 leek, soaked, rinsed, and finely sliced
6 cloves garlic, minced
2 teaspoons arrowroot powder
1 cup (250 ml) dry white wine
4 cups (1 liter) low sodium chicken broth
3 cups (100 g) baby spinach
1 cup (30 g) fresh parsley
1 teaspoon sea salt
¾ teaspoon freshly ground black pepper
½ cup (125 ml) canned full-fat coconut milk
12 to 14 large prawns, peeled and deveined
¼ cup (65 ml) coconut cream
Zest of 1 lemon
2 tablespoons fresh thyme, finely chopped

Place a large cast-iron pot or soup pot over medium heat. Add the butter and 2 tablespoons of the olive or coconut oil. Once hot, add the leek. Cook for 5 minutes, stirring often with a wooden spoon. Add the garlic and cook for 30 seconds. Sprinkle in the arrowroot powder and mix well.

Slowly add the white wine and chicken broth, stirring constantly, then lower the heat and simmer for 10 minutes.

Add the spinach, parsley, salt and pepper. Cook for another 3 minutes, then remove from heat.

Puree with an immersion blender, or transfer to a blender and puree, then return to pot.

Add the coconut milk and continue to simmer as you prepare the prawns.

Heat the remaining 1 tablespoon olive or coconut oil in a large skillet over high heat. Add the prawns and sauté for 3 minutes, then remove from heat.

With a whisk or eggbeater, whip the coconut cream for about 3 minutes, until firm.

Taste the soup and adjust seasonings if necessary, then ladle the soup into bowls. Carefully place 2 prawns in each bowl. Add a scoop of coconut cream, then top with lemon zest and a pinch of fresh thyme.

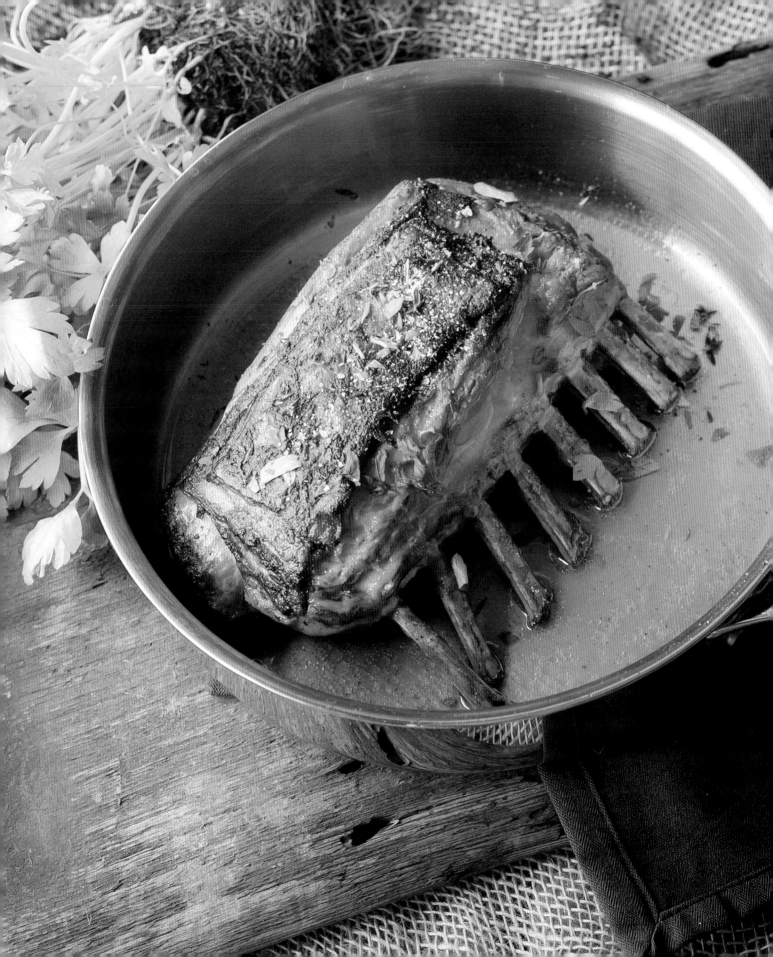

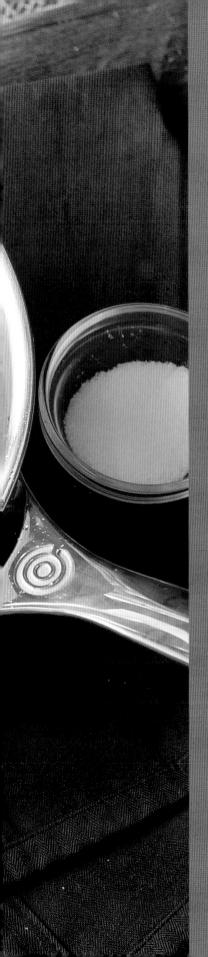

MEAT & POULTRY MAIN COURSES

These dishes are my mainstays for weeknight meals, as well as dinner parties and family gatherings. Most have a Tuscan influence, and of course all of them adhere to Paleo standards. Many of these recipes can be made in advance; they're also easy to prepare and don't require hard-to-find ingredients. Check the ingredients listings beforehand and keep your pantry stocked with the essentials, and you'll have no trouble wowing friends and family with your repertoire of Paleo Italian specialties.

As you cook, enjoy your time in the kitchen. Always have a bottle of good red or white wine close by so you can pour yourself a glass and add some to the foods you're preparing.

ROLLED, STUFFED CHICKEN IN PARCHMENT PAPER

My husband and took a cooking class in Tuscany where we learned about roasting chicken in parchment paper. It was an amazing experience, and I had to create my own Paleo version to share.
If deboning a chicken is daunting, ask your butcher to do it.

 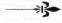

PREP TIME: 20 MINUTES
COOK TIME: 1 HOUR, 30 MINUTES
SERVES: 4

STUFFED CHICKEN

1 tablespoon olive oil

4 oz (125 g) pancetta, diced

1 whole chicken (about 3¾ lbs / 1.7 kg), deboned

2 teaspoons sea salt

1 teaspoon freshly ground black pepper

3 cups (100 g) fresh baby spinach leaves

3 cloves garlic, minced

1 teaspoon dried parsley

1 teaspoon dried thyme

½ teaspoon dried red pepper flakes (optional)

1 cup (250 ml) chicken broth

MUSHROOM GRAVY

2 cups (150 g) mushrooms, sliced

1 cup (250 ml) chicken broth

½ cup (125 ml) white wine (optional)

½ teaspoon sea salt

½ teaspoon freshly ground black pepper

½ teaspoon dried thyme

2 teaspoons arrowroot powder

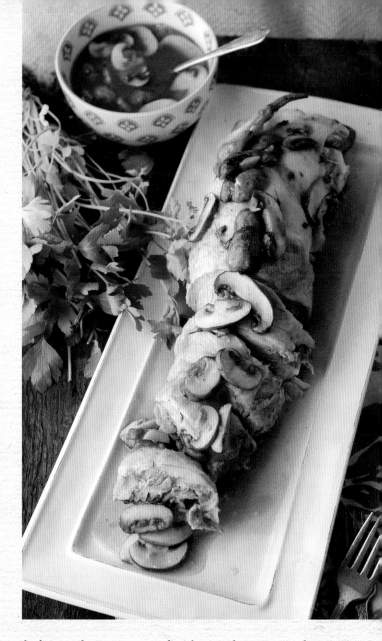

MAKING THE ROASTED CHICKEN

Place a skillet over medium heat. Add the olive oil. When hot, add the diced pancetta and cook for about 8 minutes, or until almost crisp. Place on a paper-towel-lined plate and set aside. Reserve pan and oil for later use. Preheat oven to 375°F (160°C).

Lay the chicken meat skin-side down in the center of a large piece of parchment paper. Season with the salt and pepper.

Spread the spinach on top of the chicken. Sprinkle the garlic, parsley, thyme and red pepper flakes, if using, on top, distributing evenly. Do the same with the pancetta.

Fold or roll the chicken, ensuring that all of the ingredients stay inside. Wrap the parchment paper around the roll and tuck the ends under, as you would a burrito.

Pour the chicken broth into a roasting pan. Lay the wrapped chicken inside. Roast in oven for 1 hour and 15 minutes, then remove it from the pan and place it on a board or platter to rest while you make the mushroom gravy.

MAKING THE MUSHROOM GRAVY

Heat the reserved skillet over medium heat. When the oil is hot, add the mushrooms and sauté for 8 to 10 minutes until they begin to soften. Set aside.

Place the roasting pan on the stove over medium heat. Add the chicken broth and wine, if using. Use a whisk to loosen the brown bits from the bottom of the pan and mix them into the liquid. Add the salt, pepper and thyme. Bring to a boil, then add the arrowroot powder and continue to whisk until the gravy thickens. Reduce the heat to low and add the sautéed mushrooms.

Unwrap the parchment and slice the chicken. Arrange the slices on a serving platter and pour mushroom gravy over.

BRICK-BAKED CORNISH GAME HENS

This is the perfect romantic dinner for two! You can use also use chicken in this recipe, but Cornish game hens are a nice size and have a delicate flavor. The idea of cooking poultry under foil-wrapped bricks is based on a Tuscan dish called pollo al mattone. *The bricks press the meat into the hot pan, making an even crust, and also helps keep it juicy.*

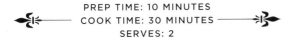

PREP TIME: 10 MINUTES
COOK TIME: 30 MINUTES
SERVES: 2

2 Cornish game hens
Grated zest of 1 lemon
1 cup (50 g) fresh parsley, finely chopped
2 tablespoons fresh rosemary, chopped
1 teaspoon sea salt
4 cloves garlic, minced
3 tablespoons olive oil, divided

Using kitchen shears, cut along both sides of the backbone of each hen; remove backbone and discard.

Using a sharp chef's knife, split each hen in half through the breast bone. Rinse the halves and pat dry with paper towels. Set aside.

Combine the lemon zest, parsley, rosemary and salt in a small bowl.

Add the minced garlic and mix well. Loosen the skin on the hens and rub seasonings under and on skin. Brush hen halves with 2 tablespoons of the olive oil.

Preheat oven to 400°F (200°C). Wrap two clean bricks in heavy-duty aluminum foil.

Heat the remaining olive oil in a large ovenproof skillet over medium-high heat. Place hen halves, skin side up, in the skillet. Cook until well-browned, about 5 minutes. Turn the hen halves over and remove from heat.

Place the foil-wrapped bricks on top of the hen halves and transfer to the oven. Bake for 25 minutes, or until a meat thermometer reads 180°F (82°C).

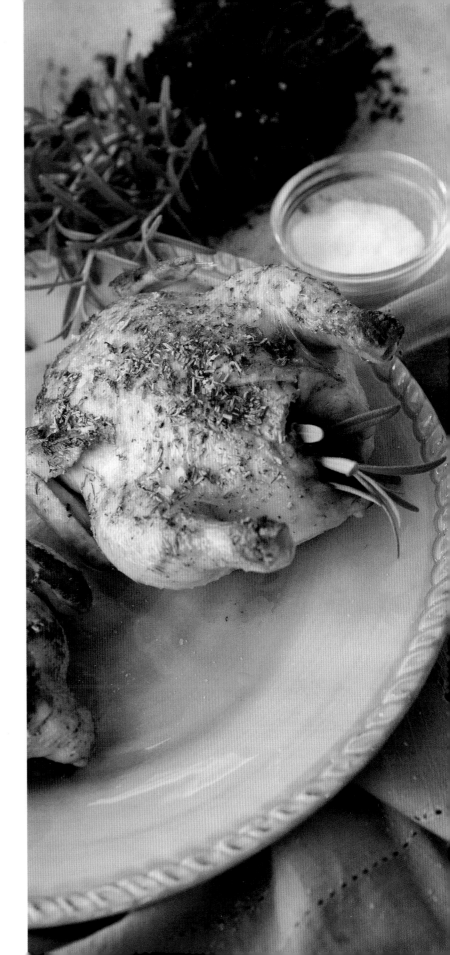

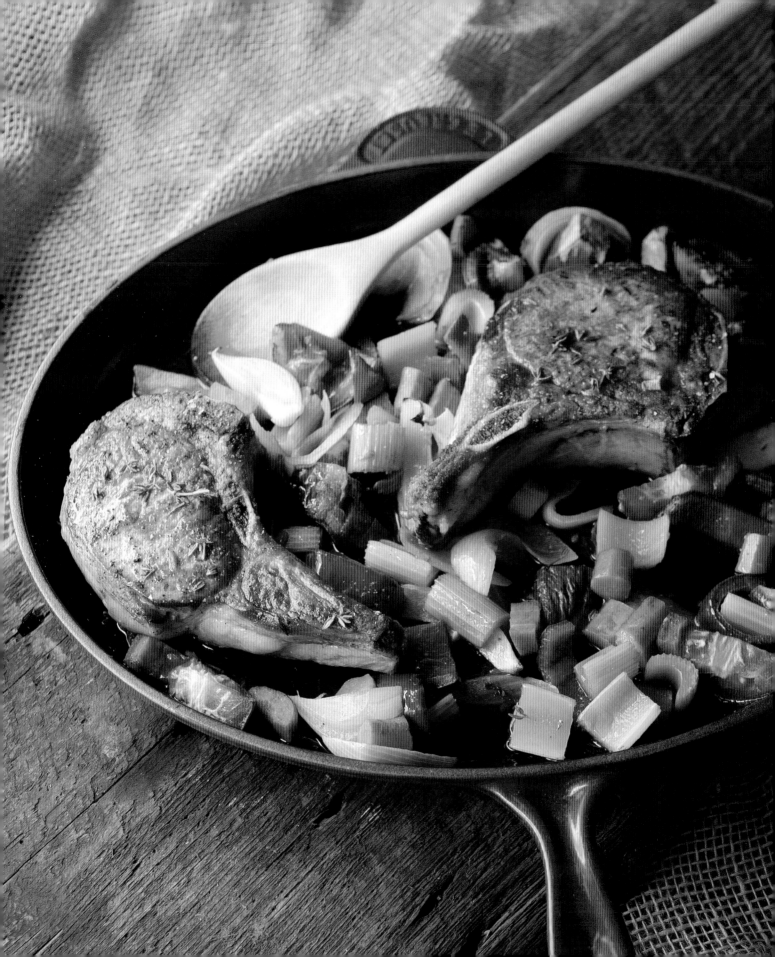

BRAISED TUSCAN PORK CHOPS

The word sofrito *appears in many Tuscan and Spanish recipes. Sofrito is a seasoning sauce made from tomatoes, onions, peppers, carrots, garlic and fresh herbs. I use it often to add depth of flavor to recipes; it complements this dish perfectly. These pork chops also go well with zucchini "noodles" (instructions to the right), spaghetti squash or grilled vegetables.*

PREP TIME: 15 MINUTES
COOK TIME: 40 MINUTES
SERVES: 4

4 thick pork chops
¼ cup (65 ml) olive oil, divided
4 plum tomatoes, chopped
1 red or green bell pepper, finely chopped
1 medium carrot, finely chopped
2 stalks celery, finely chopped
1 small yellow onion, finely chopped
3 cloves garlic, finely chopped
1 teaspoon sea salt
½ teaspoon freshly ground black pepper
¼ teaspoon dried red pepper flakes (optional)
½ teaspoon dried thyme
½ teaspoon dried basil
½ cup (125 ml) white wine or chicken broth

Separate the pork chops and lay them out on a large platter or work board.

Heat a large sauté pan or cast-iron skillet over medium-high heat. (The pan should be large enough to fit all 4 pork chops comfortably.) When hot, add 1 to 2 tablespoons of the olive oil. Once the oil is very hot, add the pork chops.

Cook the pork chops until brown on both sides, about 5 minutes per side. Remove from pan, cover with foil and set aside.

Reduce the heat to medium and add another 1 to 2 tablespoons of the olive oil.

Once hot, stir in the tomatoes, pepper, carrot, celery, onion and garlic. Cook for 3 minutes; stirring frequently with a wooden spoon.

Add the salt, pepper, red pepper flakes, thyme and basil. Mix to combine.

Return the pork chops to the pan and top with the tomato mixture.

Pour in the wine or broth, then cover, reduce heat to low and simmer for 30 minutes.

Making Zucchini "Noodles" (optional)

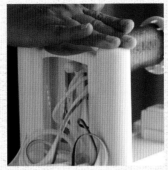

Set up a "spiralizer" kitchen tool and insert a zucchini.

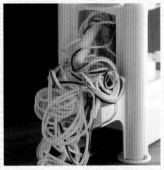

Rotate the zucchini as the "noodles" are produced.

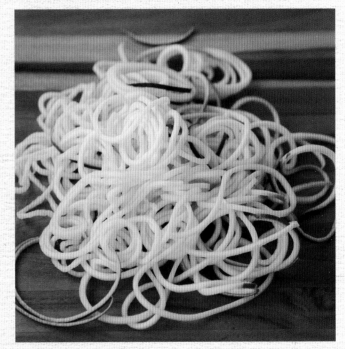

Stir-fry the "noodles" in olive oil for one minute.

RACK OF LAMB MARSALA

Using rack of lamb for this dish makes for an impressive centerpiece; however, boneless lamb may be used instead. And do use fresh herbs if you can get them—they add a completely different dimension that makes for an extra-special meal.

 PREP TIME: 15 MINUTES
COOK TIME: 30 MINUTES
SERVES: 4

2 racks of lamb, French trimmed
½ cup (145 g) chopped fresh parsley
¼ cup (7 g) fresh thyme leaves
1 tablespoon chopped fresh rosemary
2 tablespoons unsalted butter, melted
Zest of 1 lemon
2 teaspoons lemon juice
1¼ teaspoons sea salt, divided
¾ teaspoon freshly ground black pepper, divided
1½ to 2 tablespoons Dijon mustard
2 to 3 tablespoons olive oil, coconut oil, or lard
½ cup (125 ml) marsala
1 cup (250 ml) lamb or chicken stock
1 tablespoon butter

Preheat oven to 350°F (175°C).

Set the lamb on a platter or work board.

In a food processor, mini chopper or blender, combine the parsley, thyme, rosemary, butter, lemon juice, lemon zest, salt and pepper. Blend until uniform.

Coat both sides of the lamb racks with the Dijon mustard, then spread the herb mixture over the exposed meat.

Heat a large skillet over medium-high heat and add the oil. Once hot, sear each rack of lamb, one at a time, for 3 minutes per side. Reserve the skillet.

Place the lamb on a baking sheet or roasting pan and roast in the oven for 15 minutes.

Return the skillet to medium-high heat. Add the marsala and the stock. Bring to a boil, then reduce the heat to medium. Cook until the liquid is reduced by half, then whisk in the butter.

Remove the lamb from the oven and transfer to a large platter. Drizzle the marsala sauce over the meat, then serve.

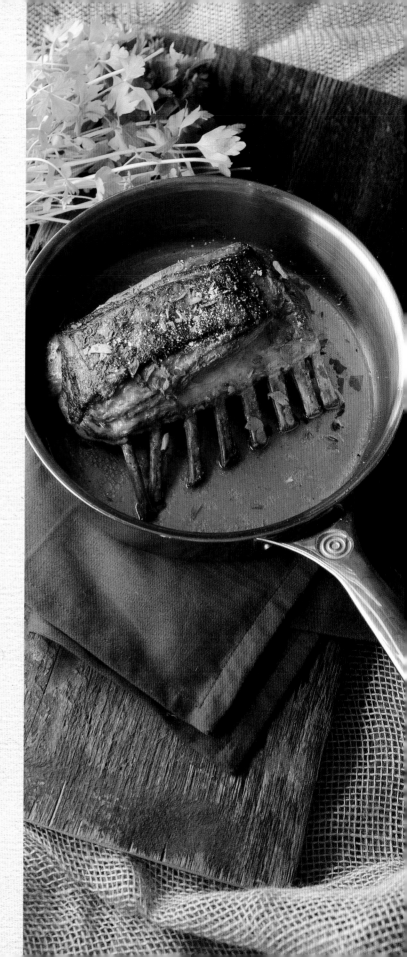

SPICY GRILLED RIBEYE WITH A FRIED EGG

Cooking ribeye with a spicy rub is already a departure from the ordinary. Fried eggs take it into a whole new realm, adding unexpected richness and texture.

PREP TIME: 10 MINUTES
COOK TIME: 15 MINUTES
SERVES: 2

2 ribeye steaks

1½ teaspoons sea salt

¾ teaspoon freshly ground black pepper

1 teaspoon chili powder

1 teaspoon cayenne pepper

1 tablespoon butter or olive oil

2 large farm eggs, at room temperature

Preheat a grill to high.

In a small bowl combine the salt, pepper, chili powder and cayenne pepper, mixing together with a fork to distribute spices evenly.

Lay the steaks on a clean work surface. Coat both sides of the steaks with the rub mixture, reserving several pinches to season the eggs.

Grill for 5 minutes per side for a medium-rare steak. Remove steaks from the grill and let rest on a platter or board for 5 to 10 minutes.

Meanwhile, prepare the eggs. Place a nonstick pan over medium heat. When hot, add the butter or oil. Crack one of the eggs into a separate bowl, removing any stray bits of shell. When the butter is hot, add the egg to the pan. Let it cook, without touching it, until the edges begin to bubble.

Cover the egg with a piece of foil and allow to cook 2 minutes more for a runny yolk and moist white, or 3 minutes for a firm white. Tilt the pan and slide the egg out of the pan and on top of a plated steak. Repeat with the other egg. Dust the eggs with the reserved rub mixture, to taste, and serve.

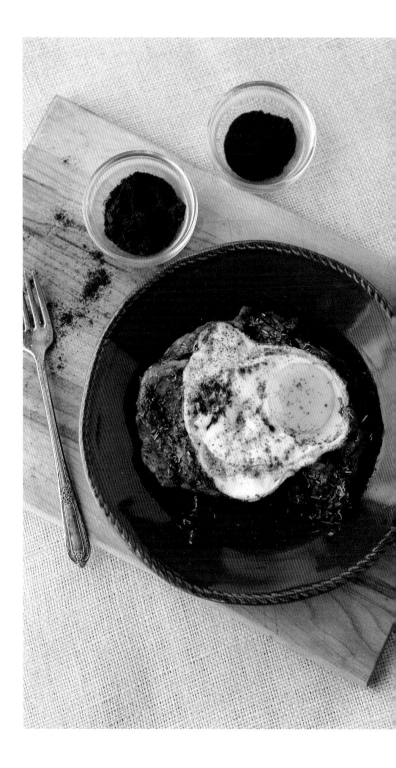

VEAL CHOPS WITH LEMON ZEST & CAPERS

The flavors in this dish are very Tuscan. For a special meal, get a good bottle of Tuscan wine to accompany it. Veal, a delicious, lean high-quality protein, is used in many Italian dishes.

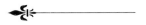 PREP TIME: 15 MINUTES
COOK TIME: 35 MINUTES
SERVES: 4

4 veal loin chops, 1¼ inch (3 cm) thick
¼ cup (65 ml) extra-virgin olive oil, divided
1¼ teaspoons sea salt
¾ teaspoon freshly ground black pepper
Zest of 1 lemon
2 tablespoons fresh thyme leaves or 2 teaspoons dried
  thyme
5 to 6 tablespoons unsalted butter
Juice of 1 lemon

Place the veal chops on a large dish or platter. Drizzle with 2 tablespoons of the olive oil and season with salt and pepper on both sides.

Season with the lemon zest and thyme. Let rest at room temperature for 20 minutes.

Preheat the oven to 400°F (200°C).

Heat a large oven-safe skillet or roasting pan over medium-high heat. Be sure the pan is large enough to hold the chops in a single layer. Melt 4 tablespoons of the butter along with the remaining 2 tablespoons of olive oil.

When the oil is very hot, add the veal chops and sear each side for about 3 minutes, turning over only once. Remove pan from heat.

Cut the remaining butter into small cubes and place on top of the veal.

Transfer the pan to the oven and roast for 15 minutes, or until an instant-read thermometer registers 160°F (72°C) for medium and 170°F (77°C) for well-done.

Squeeze the lemon juice over the veal before serving.

CINDY'S NOTE

Meat will continue to cook after it comes out of the oven. If you plan on letting the veal sit for a few minutes, remove it from the oven when the temperature is a few degrees below the final desired temperature.

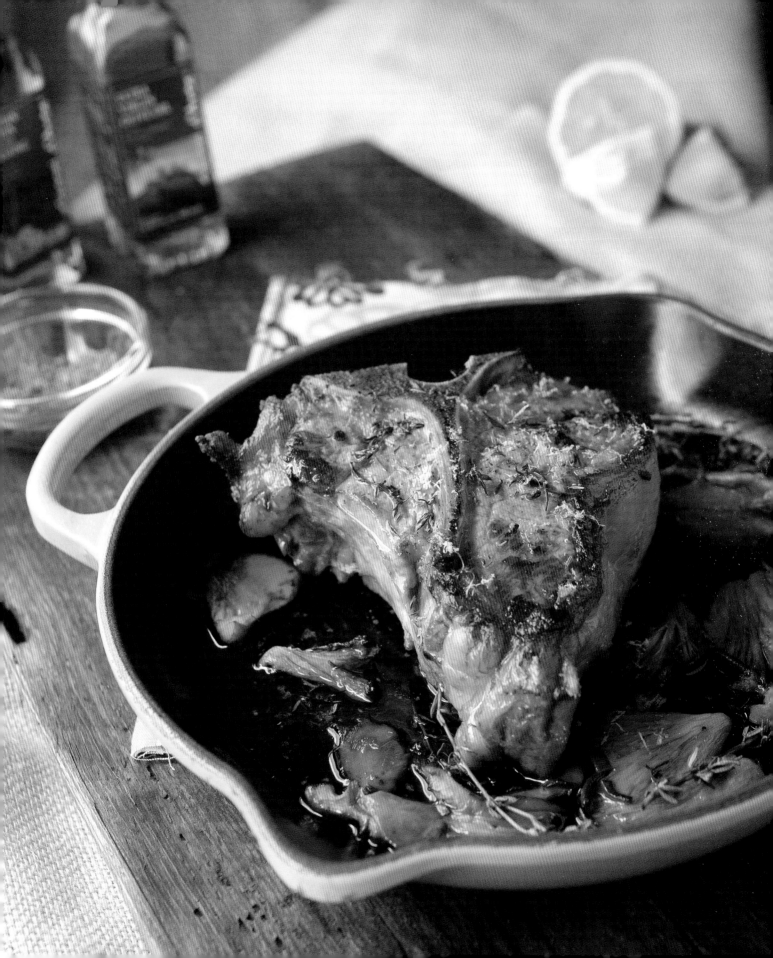

OSSO BUCO

Osso Buco is a traditional Italian meal for a Sunday dinner. The meat is slow cooked all day, infusing the house with a tempting aroma. The gremolata adds great zing and textural contrast. You can add dried red pepper flakes or diced jalapeño if you like your Osso Buco a little spicy.

When you're buying the veal shanks, let the butcher know how many servings you want to make. You may be able to get the right size for one serving per person.

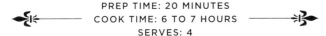

PREP TIME: 20 MINUTES
COOK TIME: 6 TO 7 HOURS
SERVES: 4

4 veal shanks, center cut

2 teaspoons of salt

1½ teaspoons freshly ground black pepper

2 tablespoons olive oil

1 tablespoon unsalted butter

1 yellow onion, sliced

3 medium carrots, sliced

4 cloves garlic, diced

2 tablespoons dried sage

1½ teaspoons of dried rosemary

One 14½-oz (400-g) can diced tomatoes

½ cup (125 ml) dry white wine

2 cups (500 ml) low-sodium chicken or beef broth

FOR THE GREMOLATA

2 cloves garlic, peeled and chopped

½ cup (10 g) fresh parsley

Zest and juice of 1 lemon

1 lemon, juiced

¾ teaspoon sea salt

Preheat oven to 225°F (105°C).

Pat the veal dry with a clean white kitchen towel, then season both sides with salt and pepper. Secure the meat around the bone by tying it with butcher's twine.

Place a large oven-safe skillet (with a cover) or a large braising pan over medium-high heat. Add the olive oil and butter.

When the oil is very hot, add the veal shanks and sear each side for about 5 minutes. (You want to create a crust on both sides).

Lower the heat to medium and stir in the onion, carrots and garlic. Cook for about 5 to 7 minutes.

Add the sage, rosemary, diced tomatoes, white wine and broth and stir well to combine all ingredients. Bring to a high simmer and cook for about 10 minutes. Taste and add more salt and

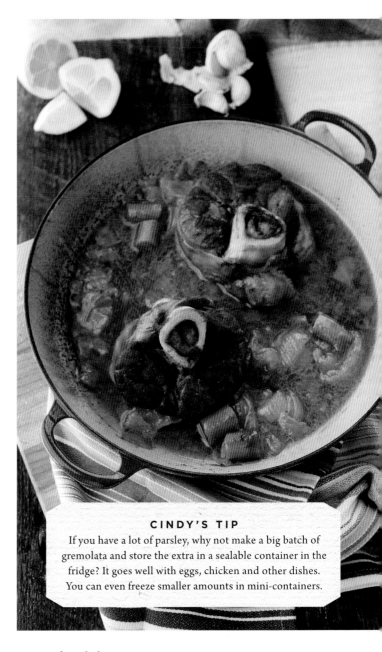

CINDY'S TIP

If you have a lot of parsley, why not make a big batch of gremolata and store the extra in a sealable container in the fridge? It goes well with eggs, chicken and other dishes. You can even freeze smaller amounts in mini-containers.

pepper if needed.

Cover and place in the oven for 5 to 6 hours.

Make the gremolata by combining all ingredients in a food processor or mini chopper and blending or processing until smooth.

Just before serving, remove the shanks from the pan, being careful to keep them from falling apart. Arrange them on a platter.

Skim off any fat from the pan with a large spoon. Pour the remaining juice into a serving bowl as a sauce to accompany the veal.

Top each piece of veal with a spoonful of gremolata.

TUSCAN BEEF TENDERLOIN

A large beef tenderloin is a dinnertime mainstay in many Italian homes—and not just as a main course. My Nana used to slice it very thick and serve as an appetizer. This tender piece of beef is perfect for any family gathering!

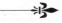

PREP TIME: 15 MINUTES
COOK TIME: 1 HOUR
SERVES: 6 TO 8

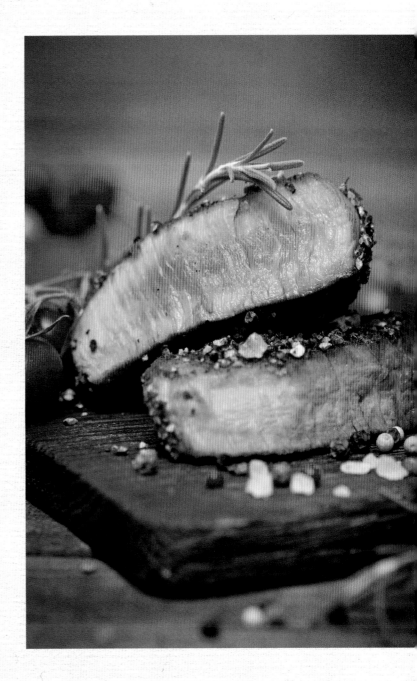

One 5-lb (2.25-kg) beef tenderloin, trimmed
¼ cup (65 ml) olive oil
1 teaspoon sea salt
¾ teaspoon freshly ground black pepper
1½ teaspoons dried basil
1 teaspoon dried parsley
1 teaspoon dried thyme
½ teaspoon dried rosemary
1 teaspoon garlic powder
2 cups (500 ml) water
4 cloves garlic, peeled and chopped
Zest and juice of 1 lemon
12 basil leaves, finely chopped
½ cup (15 g) fresh parsley, chopped
⅓ cup (75 ml) extra-virgin olive oil

Set the beef tenderloin on a large platter and drizzle the olive oil over it.

In a small bowl, combine the salt, pepper, basil, parsley, thyme, rosemary and garlic powder. Rub the mixture all over the beef, then cover and let sit for 30 minutes.

Preheat oven to 400°F (200°C).

Add the water and garlic to the bottom of a roasting pan. Place the beef on top.

Roast for 30 to 35 minutes, or until the center of the beef reaches 130°F (72°C). Remove from the oven, and tent with foil for 15 minutes before serving.

Combine lemon zest and juice, basil, parsley and extra-virgin olive oil in a small bowl. Drizzle this mixture over the beef before slicing.

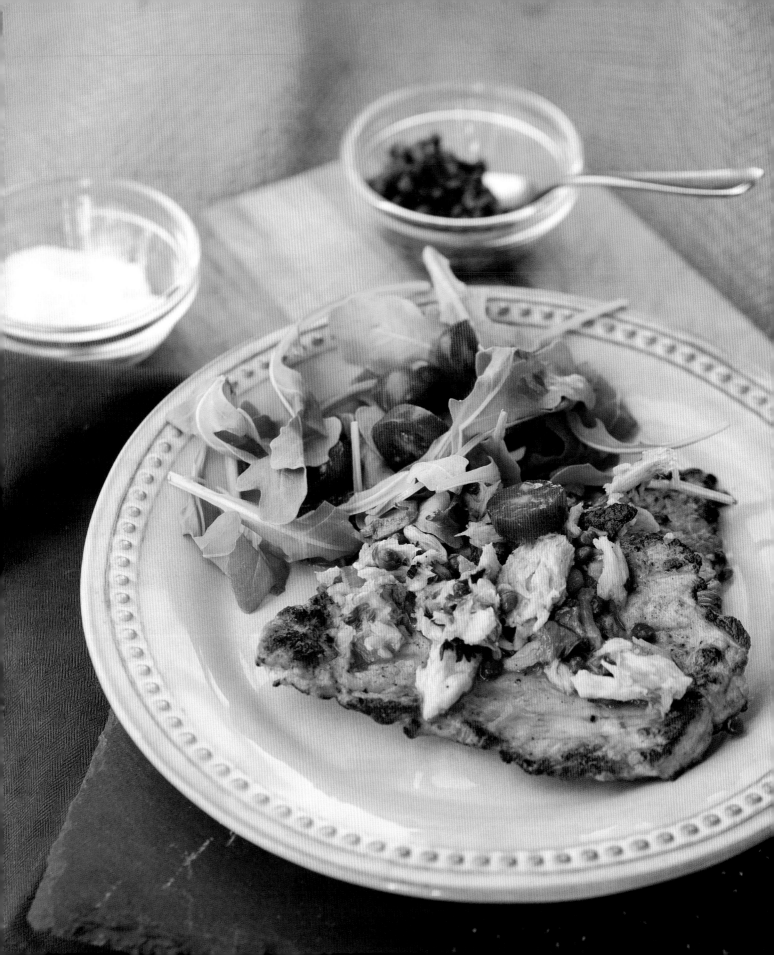

VEAL MEDALLIONS WITH TUNA & CAPER SAUCE

The tuna and capers are a great foil for the thin veal medallions. This is a real authentic Italian dish that we make again and again at our house.

PREP TIME: 15 MINUTES
COOK TIME: 25 MINUTES
SERVES: 2

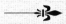

Four 4-oz (100-g) veal medallions, ½ in (1.25 cm) thick

3 tablespoons olive oil, divided

1 tablespoon unsalted butter

2 shallots, minced (about ½ cup / 50 g)

½ cup (125 ml) dry white wine

½ cup (125 ml) chicken broth/stock

One 6-oz (170-g) can tuna (chunk or solid in olive oil), drained

1 large clove garlic, finely chopped

Zest and juice of 1 lemon

3 tablespoons extra-virgin olive oil

1½ teaspoons sea salt, plus more for seasoning the veal

¾ teaspoon freshly ground black pepper, plus more for seasoning the veal

2 tablespoons capers, drained

¼ cup (5 g) fresh flat-leaf parsley, chopped

CINDY'S NOTE

If you'd rather have a warm sauce for the veal, you can add the tuna mixture to the pan with the veal in step 7 and simmer them together.

Season both sides of the veal lightly with salt and pepper and set aside on a platter.

Place a very large skillet or braising pan over medium-high heat. Add 2 tablespoons of the olive oil, along with the butter.

When the butter is bubbling but has not yet begun to brown, add the veal medallions to the pan. Cook for 3 minutes, then turn over and cook for 2 minutes more. Transfer the meat to a platter and tent with foil.

Reduce heat to medium-low and add the remaining 1 tablespoon olive oil. Once hot, add the shallots and cook, stirring, for about 4 to 5 minutes.

Add the wine and continue to cook, scraping up any browned bits from the bottom of the pan with wooden spoon, for 3 to 4 minutes, or until the liquid is almost gone.

Increase heat to medium. Add the chicken broth and simmer until reduced by half, about 4 or 5 minutes.

Return the veal medallions to the skillet and simmer for 1 minute, turning once. Transfer the veal and sauce to a platter or individual plates.

Put the tuna in a bowl and break it into bite-size pieces with a fork.

Add the garlic, lemon zest, lemon juice, olive oil, salt, pepper and capers, stirring gently to combine.

To serve, top the veal with the tuna and caper sauce.

CHICKEN SCALOPPINE IN LEMON-CAPER SAUCE

This easy dish can be a lovely romantic dinner for two or a quick dish for a family dinner. Like many Italian dishes, this one is very simple yet extremely flavorful.

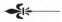

PREP TIME: 15 MINUTES
COOK TIME: 30 MINUTES
SERVES: 2

1 lb (500 g) chicken scallopine

1½ teaspoons sea salt

1 teaspoon freshly ground black pepper

3 tablespoons olive oil, divided

3 tablespoons unsalted butter or ghee, divided

2 cloves garlic, minced

1 tablespoon capers, drained

½ cup (125 ml) dry white wine

1 cup (250 ml) low sodium chicken broth

2 tablespoons fresh parsley, chopped

1 tablespoon fresh lemon juice

Place the chicken on a poultry-safe board and season with salt and pepper.

Heat a large skillet over medium heat. Once hot, add 1 tablespoon each of the oil and the butter or ghee.

When the butter is hot, add as much chicken as will fit on the pan without crowding and sear for 2 to 3 minutes on each side. When finished, set aside on a plate tented with foil. Cook the rest of the chicken in batches, heating additional oil and butter as needed each time.

Once all of the chicken is out of the pan, add the garlic. Return the chicken to the pan and add the capers.

Pour in the wine and broth and let simmer for 3 to 5 minutes to reduce the sauce.

Top with fresh parsley and lemon juice before serving.

CINDY'S NOTE
Be sure the pan is very hot before you add the chicken so that the meat sears well. The combination of oil and butter browns the chicken nicely without the need to dredge it in flour.

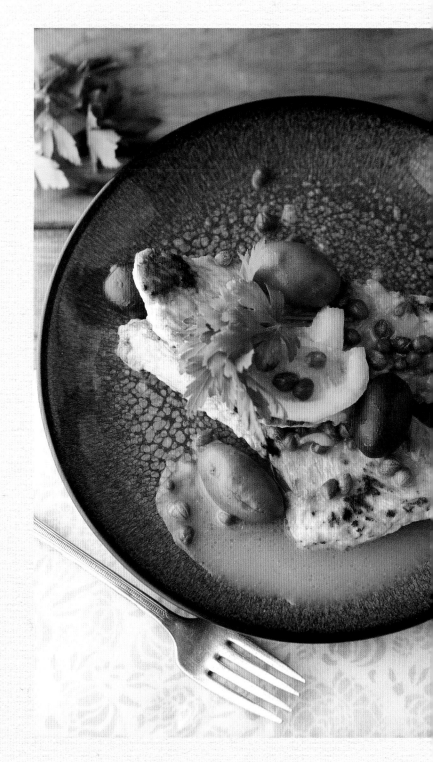

ACORN SQUASH STUFFED WITH ITALIAN CHICKEN LOAF

This is one of those comfort foods that seem to make everyone happy in autumn. I often serve it in individual bowls so everyone can enjoy their own stuffed squash half. While the acorn squash tastes fantastic with ground chicken, it's just as good with ground turkey, beef or pork.

 PREP TIME: 20 MINUTES
COOK TIME: 1 HOUR
SERVES: 2 AS A MAIN DISH,
OR 4 AS A SIDE DISH

3 tablespoons melted coconut oil, or olive oil, divided

2 medium acorn squash

1½ lbs (750 g) ground chicken

1 medium yellow onion, diced

1 small red bell pepper, diced

1 medium carrot, shredded

2 or 3 cloves garlic, minced

1 large egg

1¼ teaspoons sea salt

¾ teaspoon freshly ground black pepper

1 teaspoon dried basil

1 teaspoon dried thyme

1 teaspoon dried parsley

¼ to ½ teaspoon dried red pepper flakes

Preheat oven to 350°F (175°C).

Brush 2 tablespoons of the coconut or olive oil on the bottom of a large roasting pan or baking dish.

Cut the squash in half and remove the seeds and pulp with a tablespoon. Place in the prepared pan.

Place the ground chicken in a large mixing bowl and set aside.

Place a skillet over medium-high heat. Add the remaining 1 tablespoon oil. When hot, add the onion, pepper and carrot and cook for 3 minutes.

Add the garlic and cook for 1 minute more, then remove from heat and let cool.

Add the egg, salt, pepper, basil, thyme, parsley and red pepper flakes to the ground chicken. Then add in cooled vegetables. Combine well with your hands, but do not overmix.

Scoop the mixture into the 4 acorn halves, distributing evenly.

Bake for 1 hour and enjoy!

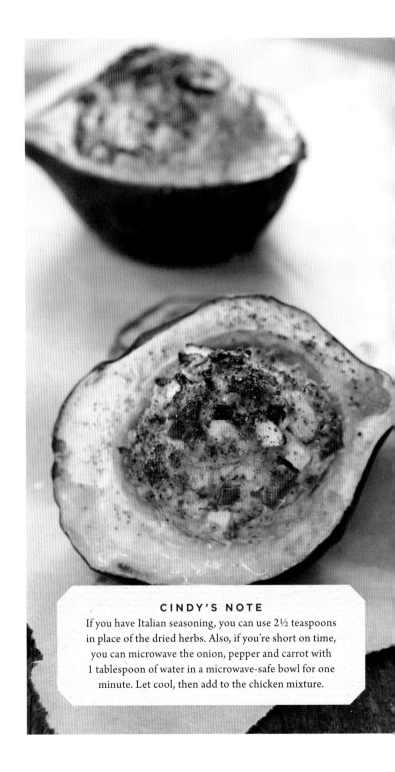

CINDY'S NOTE
If you have Italian seasoning, you can use 2½ teaspoons in place of the dried herbs. Also, if you're short on time, you can microwave the onion, pepper and carrot with 1 tablespoon of water in a microwave-safe bowl for one minute. Let cool, then add to the chicken mixture.

ROAST PORK TENDERLOIN WITH GREENS & HERBS

Roasting pork tenderloin heightens the natural flavors; adding the greens and herbs makes this meal extra-special. You should allow the pork tenderloin to marinate overnight or for at least 6 hours for best results.

 PREP TIME: 20 MINUTES, PLUS AT
LEAST 6 HOURS FOR MARINATING
COOK TIME: 45 MINUTES
SERVES: 4

One 3- to 4-lb (1.35- to 1.8-kg) boneless pork tenderloin, tied with kitchen twine

¼ cup (65 ml) olive oil, divided

6 to 8 cloves garlic, chopped

2 to 3 green onions (scallions), green and white parts, finely chopped

6 to 7 sprigs rosemary

¼ cup (5 g) fresh thyme leaves

1½ teaspoons fennel seeds

Zest and juice of 1 lemon

1 fennel bulb, cleaned and chopped

2 celery stalks, chopped

2 to 3 medium carrots, chopped

1 yellow onion, sliced

1½ teaspoons sea salt, plus more for seasoning the pork

1 teaspoon freshly ground black pepper, plus more for seasoning the pork

¾ cup (185 ml) white wine

4 cups (1 liter) low-sodium chicken broth/stock, divided

2 tablespoons unsalted butter

1 teaspoon arrowroot powder

Place the tenderloin on a poultry-safe board. Rub 2 tablespoons of the olive oil over the pork, then season with salt and pepper.

Strip the rosemary leaves from the stem and combine the garlic, scallions, rosemary leaves, thyme, fennel seeds, lemon zest and lemon juice in a food processor or mini-chopper. Process until smooth. Coat the tenderloin with the mixture.

Place the pork in a roasting pan or on a platter. Cover and refrigerate overnight, or at least 6 hours.

About an hour before serving, preheat oven to 325°F (160°C).

Place the tenderloin on a rack in a roasting pan. Arrange the fennel, celery, carrots and onions around the pork. Drizzle the remaining 2 tablespoons of olive oil over the vegetables and add the salt and pepper.

Add the wine and chicken broth to the roasting pan.

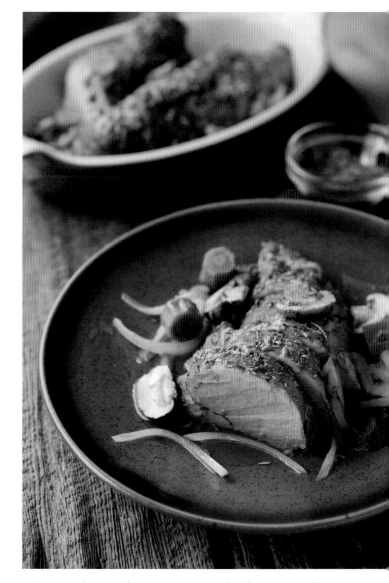

Roast until a meat thermometer inserted in the center reads 153°F (68°C), about 45 minutes.

Transfer the pork and vegetables to a platter and tent with foil. Let it rest while you make the gravy; the roast will continue cooking.

If your roasting pan is stove-safe, place it over medium heat and bring the liquid to a boil while whisking; otherwise pour the liquid into a skillet and whisk. Add the butter and continue whisking until the butter melts. Whisk in the arrowroot powder and cook until the gravy thickens.

Slice the tenderloin and arrange on a serving platter. Serve the gravy in a bowl alongside or pour it over the sliced pork.

TUSCAN TURKEY BURGERS

To evoke authentic Tuscan flavors, remember a few key elements. Include a blend of fresh vegetables and herbs, and lightly sauté your ingredients to bring out their flavors and textures. This will help you create properly seasoned Tuscan dishes every time.

I prefer the taste of ground turkey to ground beef or pork in this Tuscan burger. The lighter flavor really allows the spices to shine through. Try adding it to a chopped salad for variety!

 PREP TIME: 15 MINUTES
COOK TIME: 15 MINUTES
SERVES: 4

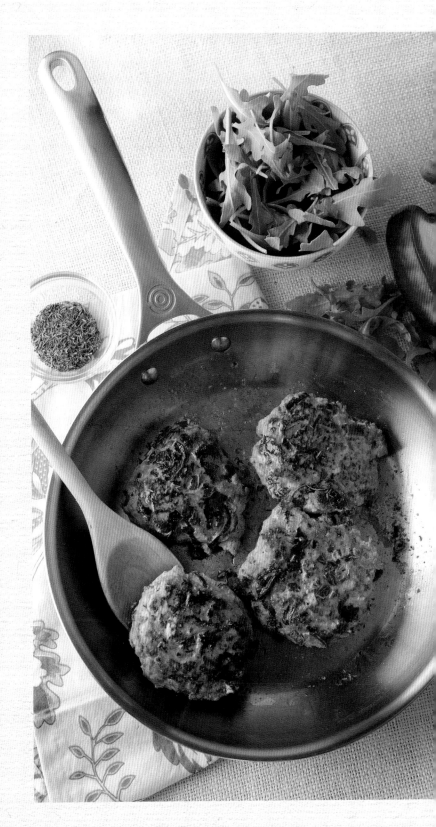

1 lb (500 g) ground turkey

1 large egg

1 teaspoon sea salt, divided

1 teaspoon freshly ground black pepper, divided

1 tablespoon olive oil

¼ cup (35 g) red pepper, diced

¼ cup (40 g) yellow onion, diced

1 clove garlic, minced

1 cup (30 g) fresh arugula or fresh baby spinach, chopped

6 leaves basil, chopped

1 teaspoon fresh thyme

¼ teaspoon dried red pepper flakes (optional)

Place the ground turkey in a large bowl. Make a well in the center and break the egg into it. Blend well with a spoon or large whisk. Season with ½ teaspoon each of the salt and the pepper and set aside.

Place a medium skillet over medium heat. Add the olive oil. Once hot, add the pepper and onion, then season with the remaining ½ teaspoon each of salt and pepper.

Continue to sauté, stirring, for 2 minutes. Add the garlic, arugula or spinach, basil, thyme and red pepper flakes, and cook for 1 minute more. Remove from heat.

Once the vegetables are cool, add them to the bowl of turkey.

Use your hands to mix all ingredients well. Form the mixture into 4 burgers.

Preheat grill to medium-high heat.

Grill burgers for 6 minutes per side, flipping once, or until a meat thermometer inserted in the center reads 160°F (72°C).

MIXED GRILL WITH ANCHOVY SAUCE

Many restaurants in Tuscany offer a mixed grill. It's a filling meal for several people. The Italian take on mixed grill is refreshingly different from those in other countries. The fresh herbs and lemon juice add a sprightly touch, and the anchovies round out the flavors of the meat very nicely.

PREP TIME: 10 MINUTES
COOK TIME: 25 MINUTES
SERVES: 4

FOR THE HERBED LEMON OIL

½ cup (125 ml) olive oil

Juice of 1 lemon

¼ cup (5 g) chopped fresh parsley

1 teaspoon dried rosemary

½ teaspoon dried thyme

½ teaspoon sea salt

½ teaspoon freshly ground black pepper

FOR THE MIXED GRILL

3–4 Italian sausages

2 boneless, skinless chicken breasts

2 strip steaks

3 tablespoons olive oil

2 teaspoon sea salt

1 teaspoon freshly ground black pepper

FOR THE ANCHOVY SAUCE

Two 2-oz (115-g) tins anchovies in olive oil, drained

2 cloves garlic

½ teaspoon dried thyme

1 tablespoon Dijon-style mustard

2 tablespoons red wine vinegar

¾ teaspoon freshly ground black pepper

1¾ cups (420 ml) extra-virgin olive oil

In small bowl combine all Herbed Lemon Oil ingredients. Stir to blend, then cover and set aside.

Preheat an outdoor grill or indoor grill pan to medium-high.

Lay the sausages, chicken and steaks on a large platter. Drizzle the olive oil over the meat and season with salt and pepper.

Grill the sausage for about 12 minutes, turning a few times. Grill the chicken for about 12 minutes. Grill the steak for 7 to 9 minutes, depending on how well done you like it. Place the cooked meat on a platter and tent with foil.

Combine all Anchovy Sauce ingredients in a food processor and pulse until smooth. Transfer to a serving bowl.

To serve, cut each sausage into thirds. Slice the chicken and the steak and arrange all the meats on a large platter. Drizzle with the Herbed Lemon Oil.

Place a bowl of anchovy sauce on the platter with a spoon for diners to help themselves.

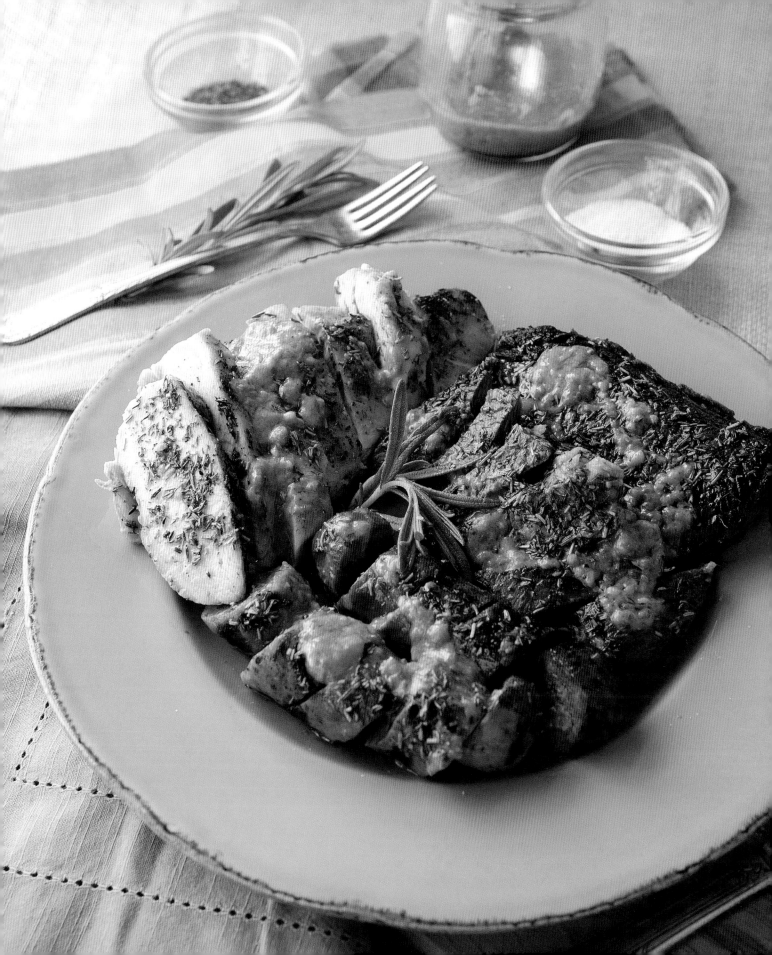

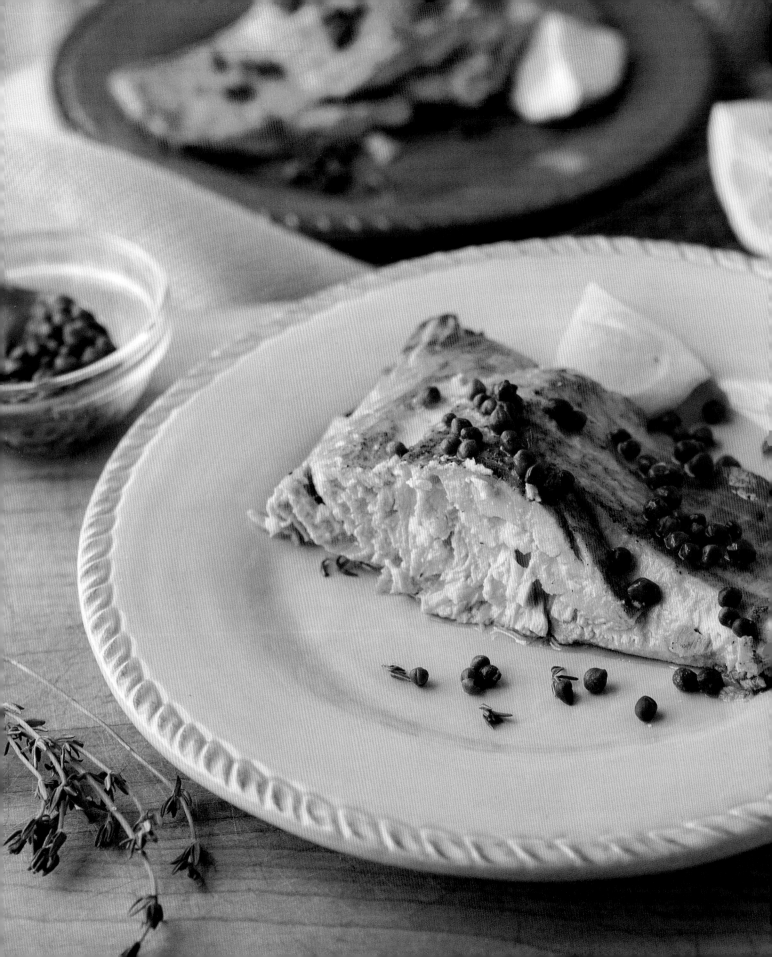

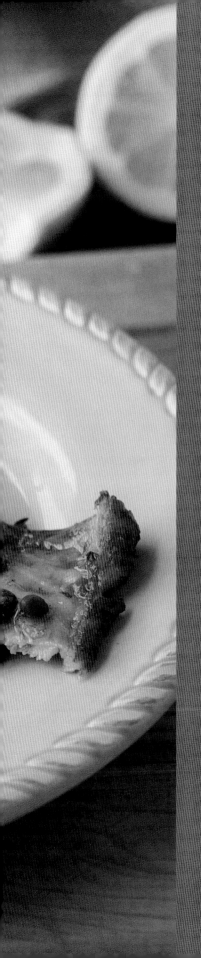

SEAFOOD MAIN COURSES

Because Italy has a lot of coastline, seafood
is a mainstay on Italian menus. My Nana was
very fond of seafood, especially cooked in a tomato
sauce with lots of garlic. I love seafood, too, and
I like coming up with new ways to prepare it. We have
a great local fish market that often inspires me.
I sometimes go in there planning to buy a certain
piece of fish, but end up coming home with something
else because they present it so beautifully. Salmon is
my absolute favorite, though—I could
eat it for breakfast, lunch, and dinner!
I'm thrilled to share these delicious Paleo Italian
seafood dishes with you.

FISH IN PARCHMENT PAPER

This recipe is a foolproof way to prepare any kind of white fish. The fish steams in the parchment paper and absorbs the flavors of the other ingredients. It's also exciting for each diner to get a papillote (parchment package) to open and enjoy.

 PREP TIME: 15 MINUTES
COOK TIME: 20 MINUTES
SERVES: 2

3 tablespoons unsalted butter, divided

1 fennel bulb, cleaned, halved lengthwise and thinly sliced

1 medium carrot, cut into thin matchstick strips

1 celery stalk, thinly sliced

2 green onions (scallions), sliced

½ teaspoon sea salt, plus more for seasoning fish

¼ teaspoon freshly ground black pepper, plus more for seasoning fish

1½ teaspoons dried tarragon

Two 6-oz (340-g) fillets Chilean sea bass or other white fish

2 teaspoons butter, divided

2 lemon slices (rounds)

Juice of 2 lemons

Preheat oven to 375°F (190°C). Line a baking sheet with foil or parchment for easy cleanup.

In a skillet over low heat add 1 tablespoon of butter, then the fennel, carrot, celery, and scallions for 7 to 8 minutes, or until soft. Stir in the salt, pepper, and tarragon. Cook for an additional 30 seconds, then remove from heat and transfer to a bowl.

Lay the fish on a platter or work board and season with salt and pepper.

Cut a piece of parchment paper about three times as big as one piece of the fish. Fold the paper in half to crease, then open and lay flat.

Place 1 teaspoon of butter on the crease. Cover it with a piece of fish and top with half of the vegetable mixture and a slice of lemon.

Bring the long edges of the paper together and fold over once. Make several small, tight folds to seal the paper, folding in the sides at the same time to create a crescent-shaped package. Place on the baking sheet and repeat with the second piece of fish and the remaining vegetables.

Bake for 15 to 20 minutes, depending on the thickness of the fish.

Place each *papillote* on a plate to serve. Have your diners open the paper to enjoy the steam and wonderful flavors, then eat the fish right out of the package!

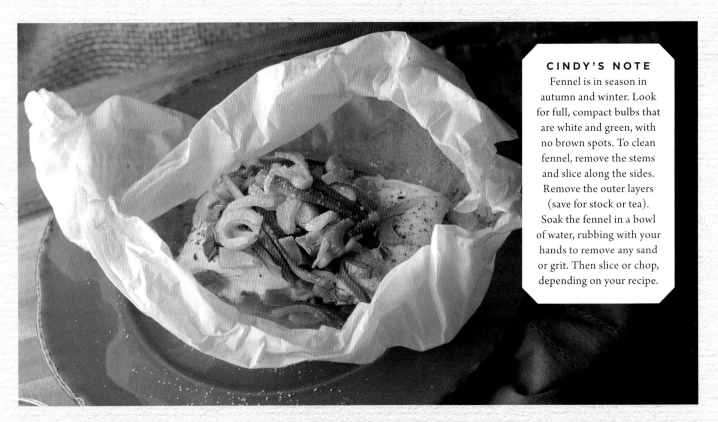

CINDY'S NOTE
Fennel is in season in autumn and winter. Look for full, compact bulbs that are white and green, with no brown spots. To clean fennel, remove the stems and slice along the sides. Remove the outer layers (save for stock or tea). Soak the fennel in a bowl of water, rubbing with your hands to remove any sand or grit. Then slice or chop, depending on your recipe.

PISTACHIO-CRUSTED COD WITH ROASTED PEPPER SAUCE

You can use any white fish in this recipe, but cod works really well. The textural contrast between the crunchy pistachios, flaky fish, and smooth sauce makes it a real winner—and the flavors combine very nicely as well!

PREP TIME: 15 MINUTES
COOK TIME: 30 MINUTES
SERVES: 2

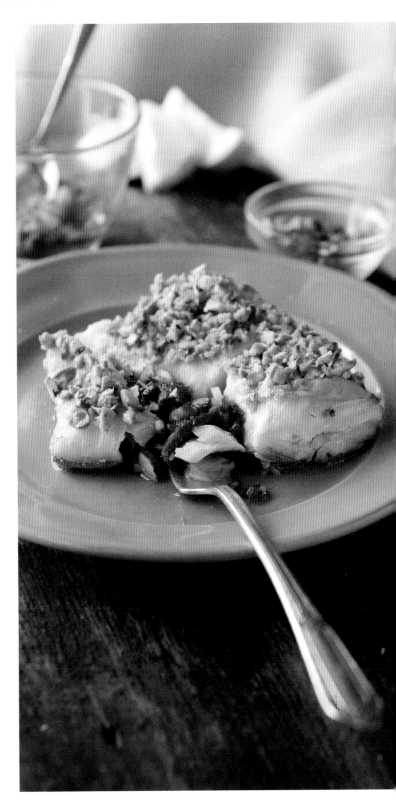

¼ cup (50 g), plus 1 tablespoon finely chopped shelled pistachios

2 cloves garlic, minced

1 teaspoon sea salt

½ teaspoon freshly ground black pepper

1 large egg

1 tablespoon Dijon mustard

One 1-lb (450-g) cod filet cut into 4 pieces

Olive oil, for drizzling

FOR THE ROASTED RED PEPPER SAUCE

1 small yellow onion, chopped

2 tablespoons chopped fresh flat flat-leaf parsley

3 jarred roasted red peppers, drained and chopped

½ cup (125 ml) low-sodium chicken broth

½ teaspoon freshly ground black pepper

Preheat oven to 400°F (200°C). Line a baking sheet with parchment paper.

Combine the pistachios, garlic, salt and pepper in a shallow dish and stir together.

Whisk the egg and Dijon mustard together in a shallow bowl.

Dip each piece of cod into the egg mixture, then roll in the pistachios and place on the prepared baking sheet. Drizzle with a little olive oil.

Bake for 12 minutes.

Combine the onion, parsley, roasted red peppers, chicken broth and pepper in a food processor and process until smooth. Pour the mixture into a saucepan and heat to warm through.

To serve, arrange the cod on a platter. Serve the warm roasted red pepper sauce in a bowl on the side or pour it over the fish.

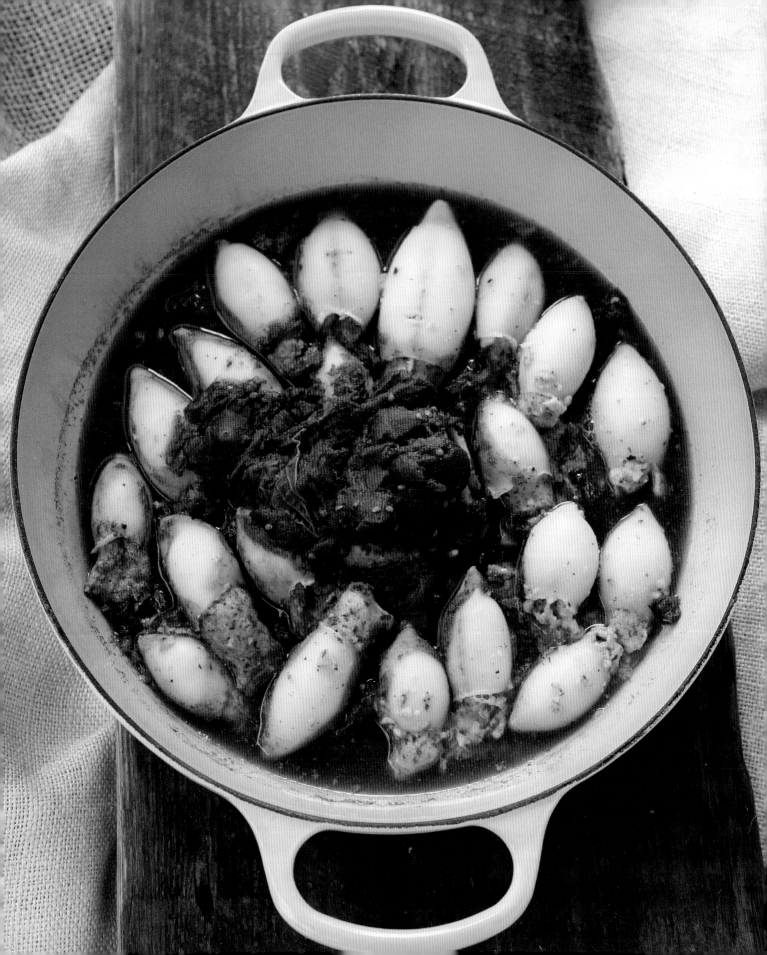

ITALIAN STUFFED SQUID

This is a very traditional Italian recipe served in many Tuscan restaurants, as well as in many Italian homes. For an authentic—but not strictly Paleo—Italian touch, add freshly grated Parmesan cheese to the stuffing mixture.

 PREP TIME: 15 MINUTES
COOK TIME: 30 MINUTES
SERVES: 4 TO 6

½ cup (125 ml) extra-virgin olive oil, divided

1 lb (500 g) whole squid, rinsed and patted dry

2 teaspoons sea salt, divided

1 teaspoon freshly ground black pepper, divided

One 15-oz (425-g) can puréed or crushed tomatoes

1 teaspoon dried thyme

2 cloves garlic, minced

¼ teaspoon dried red pepper flakes, (optional)

½ cup (10 g) almond meal

¼ cup (5 g) chopped fresh basil

¼ cup (5 g) chopped fresh flat-leaf parsley

3 cloves garlic, minced

2 large eggs

Preheat oven to 350°F (175°C).

Coat the bottom of a large baking dish with about 2 tablespoons of the olive oil.

Season the squid with 1 teaspoon of the sea salt and ½ teaspoon of the freshly ground pepper.

Combine the tomatoes, thyme, remaining 1 teaspoon sea salt, remaining ½ teaspoon pepper, garlic and red pepper flakes in a small saucepan over medium heat. Bring to a simmer.

In a medium mixing bowl, combine the almond meal, basil, parsley, garlic and eggs. Stir well to blend.

Transfer the filling mixture to a one-gallon plastic resealable bag. Cut off one corner of the bag to make a 2-inch (5-cm) hole. Push the mixture down to the bottom of the bag.

Squeeze the mixture out of the hole to fill each squid. Arrange the squid in an even layer inside the baking pan.

Pour the tomato sauce over the stuffed squid and bake for 25 to 30 minutes, or until tender.

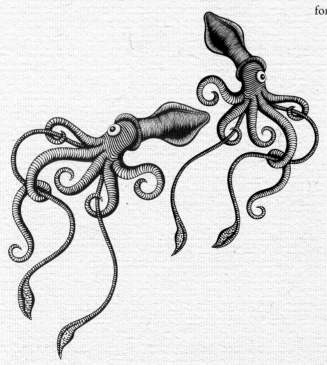

MUSSELS WITH HERBS & RED SAUCE

Mussels are a popular appetizer or snack in Italy, and they're prepared in any number of ways. My Nana sometimes prepared a pan of mussels in red sauce for a late afternoon meal, placing the pan on the table for everyone to help themselves. This dish is a perfect leisurely meal for an informal gathering of friends.

 PREP TIME: 10 MINUTES
COOK TIME: 10 MINUTES
SERVES: 4

1 tablespoon olive oil
2 cloves garlic, minced
¼ teaspoon dried red pepper flakes
½ cup (125 ml) dry white wine
One 15-oz (425-g) can diced tomatoes
2 lbs (1 kg) mussels, scrubbed

Place a large cast-iron pot over medium heat. Add the olive oil. Once hot, add the garlic and red pepper flakes. Stir with a wooden spoon for 30 seconds.

Add the wine and the diced tomatoes and bring the sauce to a boil.

Add the mussels. Cover and let cook for 6 to 8 minutes, or until the mussels open. Any mussels that do not open should be discarded.

Transfer mussels to a large bowl or bring to the table to serve right out of the pan.

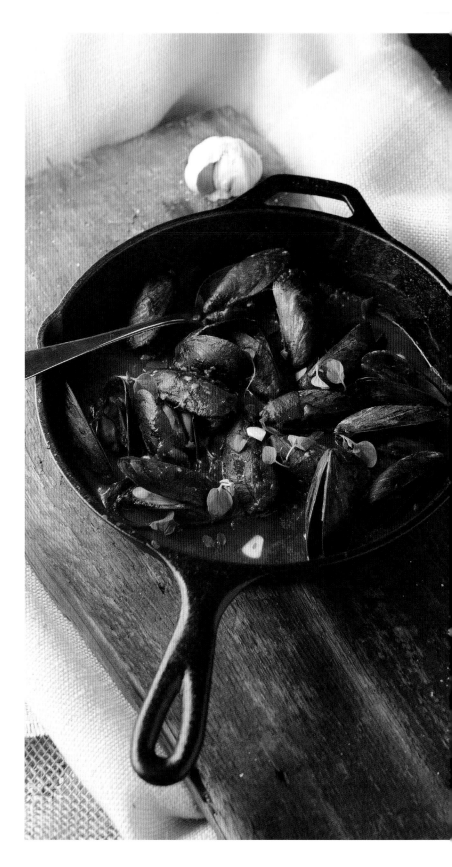

SWORDFISH WITH EGG-PLANT CAPONATA

The swordfish and eggplant are combined to brilliant effect in this dish. Caponata does take some time to make, but the results are more than worth the effort.

PREP TIME: 10 MINUTES
COOK TIME: 10 MINUTES
SERVES: 4

2 cups (450 g) prepared Eggplant Caponata (page 133, sausage omitted)
¾ cup (95 g) green olives, chopped
1 anchovy fillet, finely chopped
1 tablespoon white wine vinegar
1 large clove garlic, finely chopped
½ teaspoon dried thyme, crumbled
Four 6-oz (680-g) swordfish steaks
Extra-virgin olive oil, for drizzling
1 teaspoon sea salt
½ teaspoon freshly ground black pepper
¼ cup (5 g) chopped fresh parsley

Combine the caponata, green olives, anchovy, white wine vinegar, garlic and thyme in a large bowl and set aside.

Preheat an outdoor grill or indoor grill pan to medium.

Drizzle the swordfish with olive oil, then season with the salt and pepper. If using an indoor grill pan, brush with oil.

Grill the swordfish for 3 to 4 minutes per side, or until cooked through.

To serve, plate each swordfish and top with Eggplant Caponata. Drizzle a little olive oil over and sprinkle fresh parsley on top.

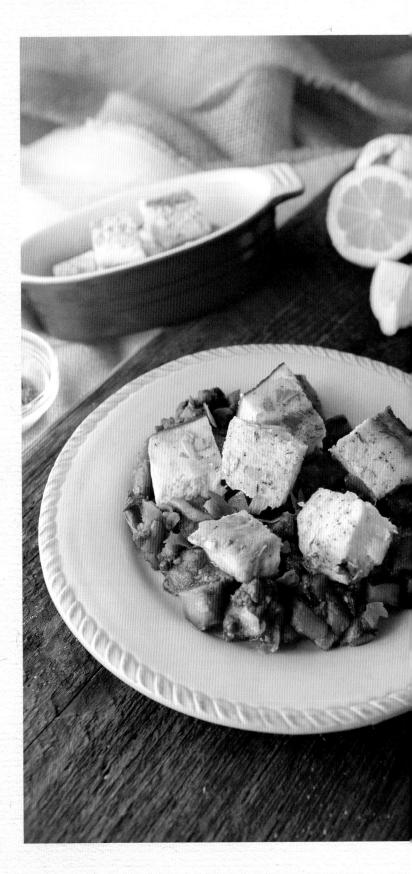

SALMON WITH LEMON, CAPERS & THYME

Lemon and capers often go together in Italian cuisine. Adding them to salmon may be an obvious choice, but it's also delicious! This is a great dish to make when you're pressed for time, as you can get it to the table in less than an hour.

PREP TIME: 10 MINUTES
COOK TIME: 25 MINUTES
SERVES: 2

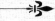

2 tablespoons extra-virgin olive oil
1 lb (500 g) salmon
1 teaspoon sea salt
½ teaspoon freshly ground black pepper
1½ teaspoons dried thyme, divided
4 or 5 thin slices lemon slices
1 tablespoon capers, drained

Preheat oven to 400°F (200°C).

Line a baking sheet or baking pan with parchment paper (for easy cleaning).

Brush a little extra-virgin olive oil on the parchment paper, then place the salmon on the paper, skin-side down.

Drizzle a little extra-virgin olive oil over the salmon, then season with the salt, pepper and 1 teaspoon of the thyme.

Top with lemon slices and the remaining ½ teaspoon dried thyme. Bake for 25 minutes.

Remove from oven and sprinkle the capers over the salmon. Serve immediately.

CINDY'S NOTE

If you cut the salmon into individual servings before baking, you can reduce the cooking time by about 5 minutes. You can also wrap the seasoned salmon and lemon in foil and cook it on a grill for 7–10 minutes.

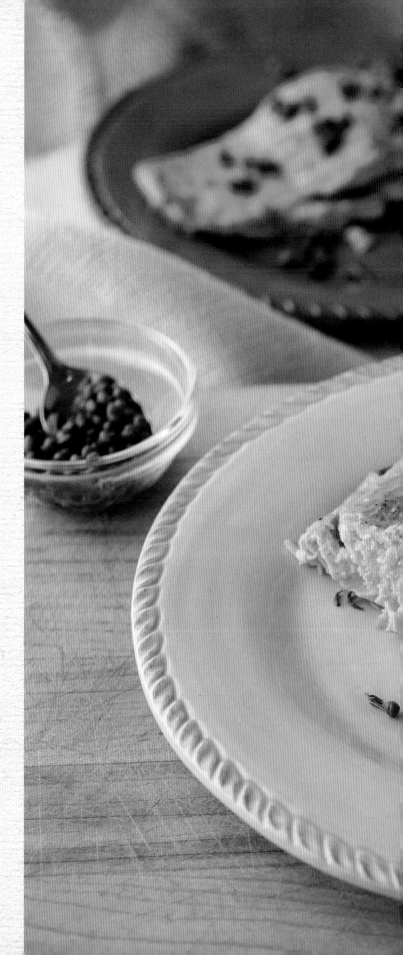

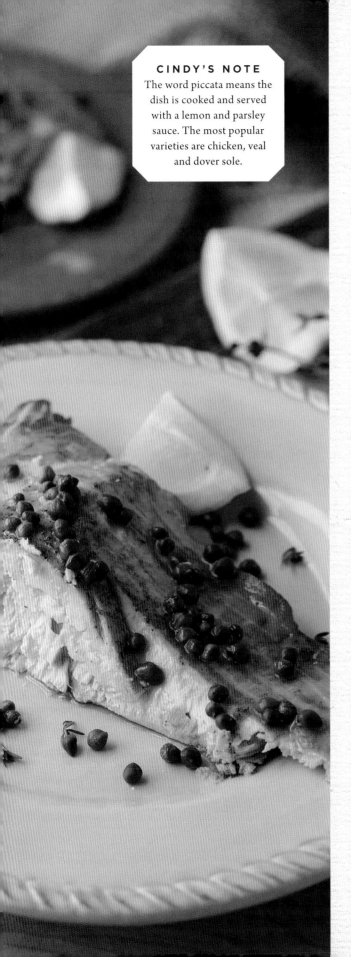

CINDY'S NOTE
The word piccata means the
dish is cooked and served
with a lemon and parsley
sauce. The most popular
varieties are chicken, veal
and dover sole.

DOVER SOLE PICCATA

I adore chicken piccata and veal piccata, but Dover Sole Piccata is my absolute favorite. It's an excellent dish to serve at a dinner party—the name alone sounds elegant, and it looks gorgeous on the table. You can make it in advance, too—just briefly sear the fish on each side, place it in a baking dish, then cover and refrigerate. Before serving, bake it for about 15 minutes in a 350°F (175°C) oven.

 PREP TIME: 10 MINUTES
COOK TIME: 15 MINUTES
SERVES: 2

1 lb (500 g) Dover sole or flounder

1¼ teaspoons sea salt

¾ teaspoon freshly ground black pepper

¼ cup (65 ml) good-quality olive oil, divided

4 tablespoons unsalted butter, divided

2 cloves garlic, minced

1 small shallot, minced

¼ cup (65 ml) white wine

¼ cup (65 ml) low-sodium chicken broth/stock

Juice of 1 lemon

4 tablespoons chopped fresh Italian parsley, divided

2 to 3 tablespoons capers, drained

Preheat oven to 150°F (65°C). Put a serving dish or platter in the oven to keep warm.

Place the fish on a large platter or work board and season both sides with the salt and the pepper.

Place a large skillet over medium heat. Depending on the size of the pan, you may need to cook the fish in batches; divide the oil and butter accordingly. Once the pan is very hot, add oil and butter for one batch of fish.

When hot, add the fish and cook for about 2 minutes on each side, or until brown. Remove from pan and place on the warmed plate in the oven. Heat the next portion of oil and butter and cook the next batch of fish. Continue until all the fish is cooked.

In the same pan, still at a medium heat, cook the garlic and shallots for 30 seconds. Deglaze the pan with the wine, then add the chicken broth. Continue to cook, whisking the liquid and scraping the bottom of the pan to pick up bits that have stuck, until the liquid is reduced by a fourth.

Add the lemon juice, 2 tablespoons of the parsley and the capers. Reduce the heat to low and return the warm fish to the pan.

Garnish with the remaining 2 tablespoons parsley and serve.

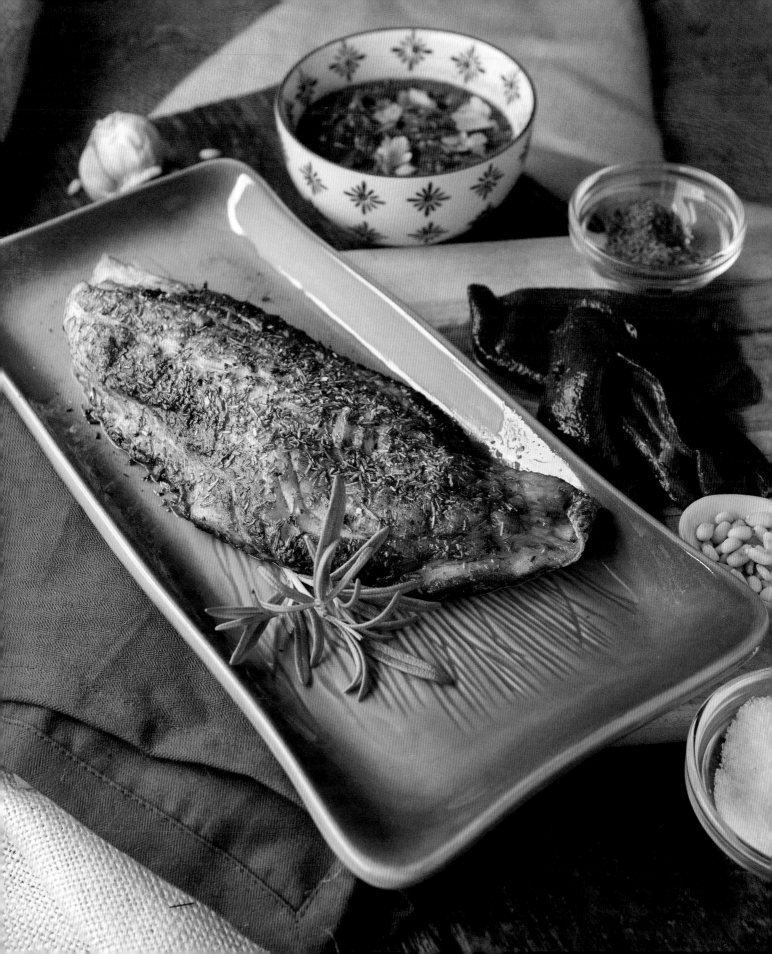

ITALIAN ROMESCO WITH RED SNAPPER

I decided on the spur of the moment to serve red snapper with a Romesco sauce for a weeknight dinner party. It turned out to be a great idea, and it was a huge hit. Though it was easy to put together, it looked as if I had spent hours preparing it.

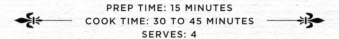

PREP TIME: 15 MINUTES
COOK TIME: 30 TO 45 MINUTES
SERVES: 4

3 roasted red peppers, jarred

2 plum tomatoes, chopped

2 cloves garlic, minced

1 teaspoon dried parsley

1¾ tablespoons balsamic vinegar

2½ tablespoons fresh rosemary or 2 teaspoons dried rosemary, divided

⅓ cup (80 ml) or more extra-virgin olive oil

Four 6-oz (175-g) fillets red snapper (1½ lbs / 700 g total)

1¼ teaspoons sea salt

¾ teaspoon freshly ground black pepper

To make the Romesco sauce, combine the roasted red peppers, garlic, parsley, vinegar, and 2 tablespoons of the fresh or 1½ teaspoons of the dried rosemary in a food processor. With the processor on low, pour ¼ cup of the olive oil in to create a thick sauce. If the sauce is too thick, add more oil a tablespoon at a time.

Place a large skillet over medium heat. Add 1 tablespoon of olive oil and the remaining rosemary.

Season the fish with the salt and pepper, then place in the hot pan. Cook for 8 to 10 minutes, turning once, until golden on both sides.

To serve, spoon Romesco sauce onto each plate and top with the cooked snapper.

CINDY'S NOTE

Instead of using jarred peppers for the Romesco sauce, why not roast your own? Preheat your oven to 400°F (200°C). Line a baking sheet with parchment or foil and place whole red peppers on it, then drizzle them with olive oil. Roast for 45 minutes, turning once halfway through. Remove from oven and immediately transfer to a large bowl. Cover the bowl with clear wrap and let stand for 20 minutes. Remove the skin layer with your fingers and take out the seeds. The peppers are ready to use!

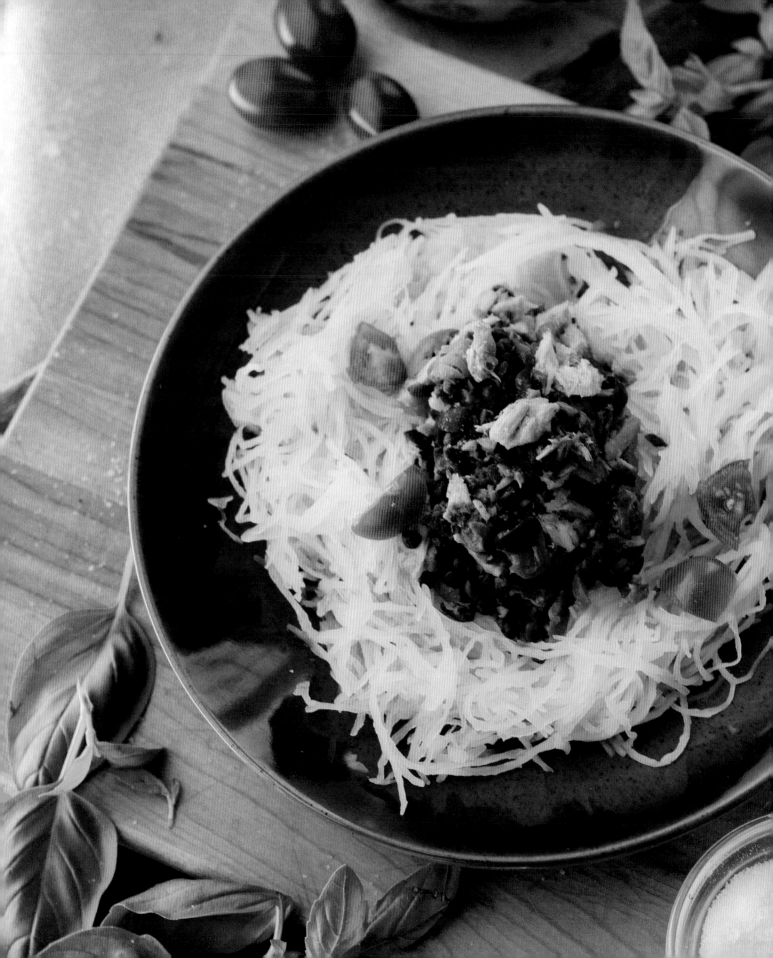

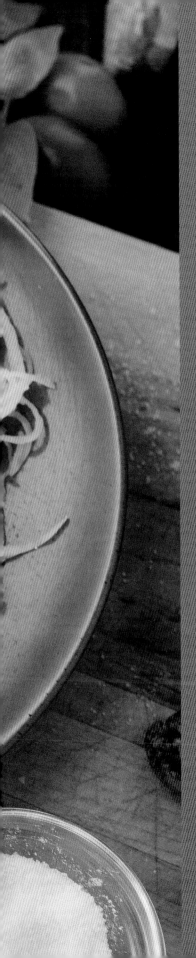

FOR PASTA LOVERS

Pasta, of course, is practically the national food of Italy.
When we were kids, it was a party when
pasta was served. My Nana would make special dishes
like spaghetti and meatballs, lasagna, or penne with
chicken and lemon sauce every Sunday. She had
a seemingly endless supply of pasta recipes, and
they were all delicious.

Today, as I enjoy the Paleo lifestyle, I have created
many "pasta" dishes that still remind me of authentic
Italian pasta dishes, but with more vibrant flavors and
fresh ingredients. I guarantee that the recipes in this
chapter will bring plenty of smiles to your dinner table!

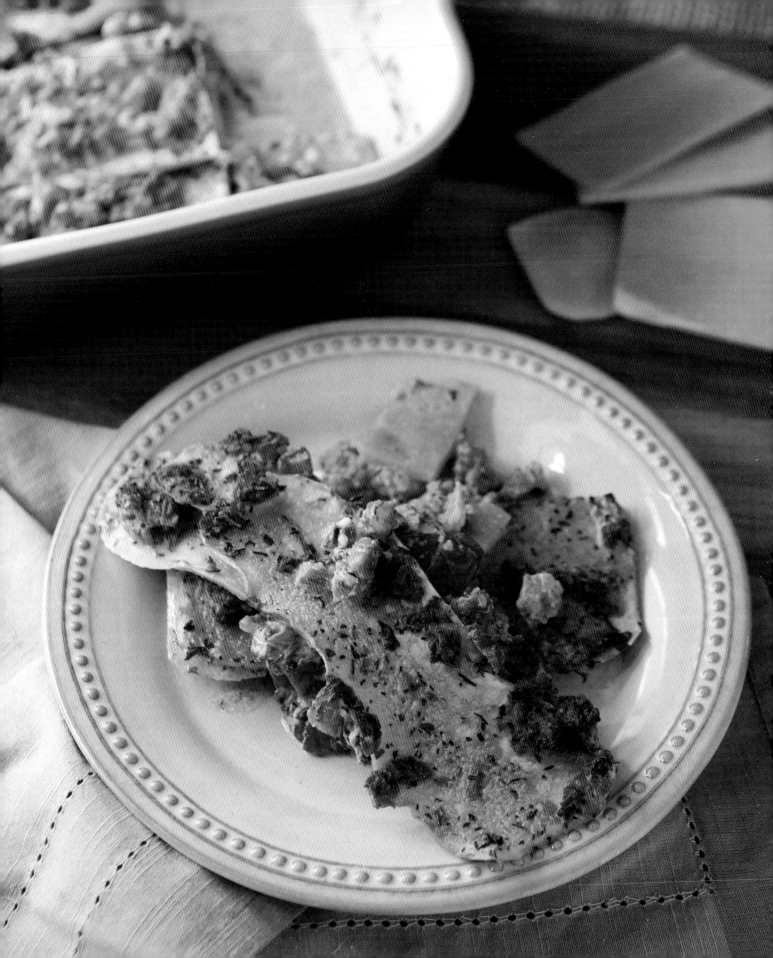

BUTTERNUT SQUASH "LASAGNA"

The butternut squash adds amazing fall flavors to this lasagna. If you have a mandoline, you can slice the squash into very thin strips for perfect lasagna "noodles." For a heartier lasagna, you can add sautéed ground beef, ground chicken or even sausage.

PREP TIME: 15 MINUTES
COOK TIME: 1 HOUR
SERVES: 4

1 large butternut squash
1 to 2 tablespoons olive oil, divided
1 teaspoon unsalted butter
½ yellow onion, diced
1 teaspoon sea salt
3 to 4 cloves garlic, chopped
1 cup (250 ml) canned full-fat coconut milk
One 15-oz (425-g) can petite diced tomatoes
1 teaspoon dried basil
1 teaspoon dried parsley
1 teaspoon dried sage
1 teaspoon freshly ground black pepper
Two 6-oz (175-g) bags baby spinach

Preheat oven to 350°F (175°C).

Cut the squash in half and remove the seeds and pulp. Use a vegetable peeler to remove the skin.

If you have a mandoline, use it to create your lasagna "noodles," or cut the squash into very thin strips with a chef's knife.

Place a large skillet over medium heat. Add 1 tablespoon of the olive oil and the butter. Add the onions and the sea salt and cook for 1 minute, then add the garlic and cook for 30 seconds.

Stir in the coconut milk, tomatoes, basil, parsley, sage and black pepper. Bring to a high simmer, then cover and remove from heat.

Microwave the spinach in the bag if possible, or place in a microwave-safe dish with 3 tablespoons of water and cook on high for 3 minutes. Squeeze the spinach to remove liquid and set aside.

Cover the bottom of a 9 x 13-inch (23 x 33-cm) baking pan with a ladleful of the tomato sauce. Cover with a layer of butternut squash strips, then spread the cooked spinach on top. Add two more scoops of the sauce to cover the spinach. Top with a layer of butternut squash strips, then pour the rest of the sauce over to cover.

Bake the lasagna, uncovered, for 45 minutes.

Remove from the oven and let rest for 5 minutes, then enjoy family-style.

How to Cut and Peel a Butternut Squash
Follow these instructions to cut and peel your butternut squash.

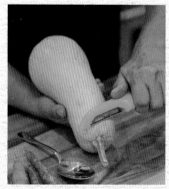

Use a peeler to carefully remove a strip of the skin from top to bottom.

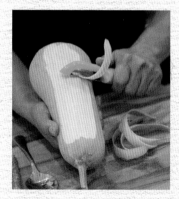

Peeling the skin of the squash.

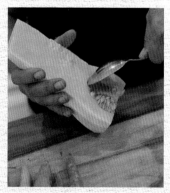

Remove the top and bottom, then slice the skinned squash in half lengthwise. Use a spoon to scoop out the seeds.

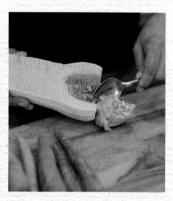

The squash is now ready to cut into thin strips.

SPAGHETTI SQUASH PUTTANESCA

Puttanesca is a Southern Italian specialty featuring a tomato sauce that typically contains olives, garlic, capers, hot pepper, and anchovies. The sauce is most often served with pasta, but it goes great with grilled chicken, too!

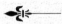

PREP TIME: 15 MINUTES
COOK TIME: 1 HOUR
SERVES: 4

1 large spaghetti squash (about 4 lbs / 1.8 kg)

2 tablespoons olive oil, plus additional for drizzling

1 small onion, finely chopped

4 cloves garlic, minced

Three 15-oz (425-g) cans plum tomatoes, (an imported Italian brand like San Marzano is best)

One 7-oz (200-g) can tomato paste

¾ cup (180 g) olives, pitted and sliced in half

2 tablespoons capers, drained

One 2-oz (115-g) tin anchovy fillets, minced

1 teaspoon dried basil

1 teaspoon dried oregano

½ teaspoon dried red pepper flakes

1 teaspoon sea salt

¾ teaspoon freshly ground black pepper

Preheat oven to 375°F (190°C).

Line a baking sheet with parchment paper. Place the spaghetti squash on the sheet and poke about 12 holes in the flesh with a long metal skewer. Bake for 50 minutes.

Place a large saucepan over medium heat and add 2 tablespoons of the olive oil. When hot, add the onion and cook for 2 minutes. Add the garlic and cook for an additional 30 seconds.

Add the tomatoes and bring to a boil, then add the tomato paste. Press the paste against the side of the pan with a spoon before stirring it in to reduce lumps. Stir about 3 tablespoons of hot water around in the can to get the last of the tomato paste, then add to the pot.

Stir in the remaining ingredients. Cover, reduce heat to low and simmer for 30 minutes.

When the squash is done, let it cool enough to touch, then slice it lengthwise and remove the seeds.

Use a fork to scrape out the flesh and separate the strands into "pasta." Transfer to a serving bowl and top with the puttanesca sauce. Drizzle a little olive oil over all before serving.

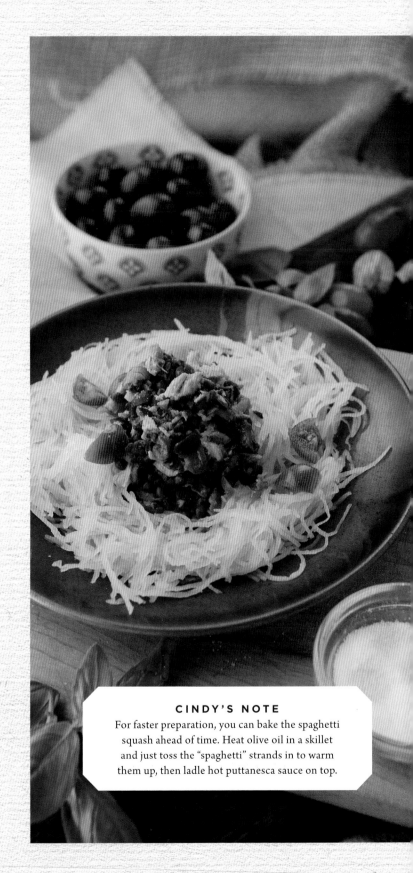

CINDY'S NOTE
For faster preparation, you can bake the spaghetti squash ahead of time. Heat olive oil in a skillet and just toss the "spaghetti" strands in to warm them up, then ladle hot puttanesca sauce on top.

SPAGHETTI SQUASH WITH A CHICKEN RAGÙ

A ragù is a thicker sauce that's generally made with meat, but chicken or mushrooms may be used instead. The longer you cook the sauce, the more intense the flavors will become. You can serve this sauce over roasted vegetables, or even over a breakfast frittata. Chicken Ragù also goes well with zucchini "noodles."

 PREP TIME: 15 MINUTES
COOK TIME: 1 HOUR
SERVES: 4

1 large spaghetti squash (about 4 lbs / 1.81 kg)

2 tablespoons olive oil or coconut oil

1 small onion, finely chopped

1 medium carrot, diced

1 celery stalk, diced

3 or 4 cloves garlic, minced

1 lb (500 g) ground chicken

One 28-oz (800-g) can crushed tomatoes

2 tablespoons tomato paste

1 teaspoon dried basil

1 teaspoon dried parsley

1 teaspoon dried oregano

1 teaspoon sea salt

¾ teaspoon freshly ground black pepper

Preheat oven to 375°F (190°C).

Line a baking sheet with parchment paper. Place the spaghetti squash on the baking sheet and poke about 12 holes in the flesh with a long metal skewer. Bake for 50 minutes.

Place a Dutch oven or large saucepan over medium heat and add the oil. Once hot, add the onions, carrot, celery and garlic. Cook for 3 minutes.

Add the ground chicken and cook about 7 minutes, until brown. Use a wooden spoon to break up the meat as it cooks.

Add the crushed tomatoes and bring the sauce to a boil. Reduce heat and add the remaining ingredients, stirring well to combine. Cover and let simmer for 20 minutes.

Taste and adjust seasonings if necessary. Continue to simmer until sauce thickens.

When the squash is done, allow it to cool enough to handle, then slice it lengthwise and remove the seeds.

Use a fork to scrape out the flesh and separate the strands into "pasta." Transfer to a serving bowl and top with the Chicken Ragù.

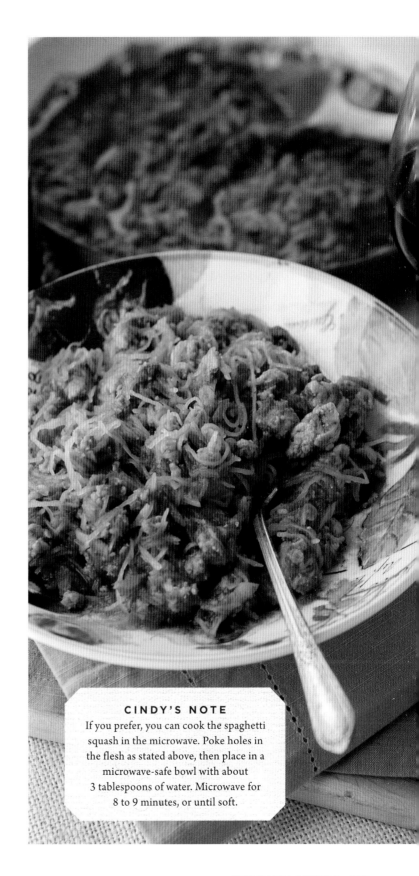

CINDY'S NOTE
If you prefer, you can cook the spaghetti squash in the microwave. Poke holes in the flesh as stated above, then place in a microwave-safe bowl with about 3 tablespoons of water. Microwave for 8 to 9 minutes, or until soft.

CAULIFLOWER "RISOTTO" WITH PORCINI MUSHROOMS & PEAS

Risotto, a specialty of northern Italy, is made from Arborio rice and cooked very slowly, with broth added a little at a time to create a creamy consistency. Nana used to pour herself a cup of coffee, grab her stool and sit at the stove for an hour making her risotto. This Paleo version, made with cauliflower instead of rice, takes less time to prepare, but duplicates the creamy texture and richness of the traditional dish.

 PREP TIME: 15 MINUTES
COOK TIME: 30 MINUTES
SERVES: 4

1 large (or 2 small) cauliflower

1¼ cups (30 g) dried porcini mushrooms

3 cups (750 ml) low-sodium chicken broth, plus more, if needed

3 tablespoons unsalted butter

1 shallot, minced

2 teaspoons sea salt

1 teaspoon freshly ground black pepper

1½ cups (200 g) frozen petite peas, thawed

1 tablespoon balsamic vinegar

1 teaspoon chopped fresh thyme

CINDY'S NOTE

Save the soaking liquid from the porcini mushrooms for use in soups or stews. You can also add a little to your risotto to give it a richer flavor.

Set up a food processor with a grater attachment. Chop the cauliflower into pieces, then shred into rice-grain-sized pieces in the food processor. (A box grater may be used if a food processor is not available.)

Pour 2 cups of boiling water into a bowl. Add the mushrooms and let sit for 20 minutes. Remove from the bowl with a slotted spoon, reserving the liquid (see note below left). Pat dry, then chop fairly finely.

Warm the broth in a medium saucepan.

Melt the butter in a Dutch oven or large pot over medium heat. Add the shallots and cook for 2 minutes. Add the cauliflower "rice," salt and pepper and let cook, stirring gently with a wooden spoon from time to time, for about 5 minutes.

Add the mushrooms and stir gently to combine. Let cook for another minute.

Add 1 cup of broth and simmer, still over medium heat, until it is absorbed into the cauliflower "rice." Repeat, adding broth 1 cup at a time, until it is all absorbed, about 15 minutes.

Add the peas, balsamic vinegar and fresh thyme. Stir and continue to cook for another 5 minutes.

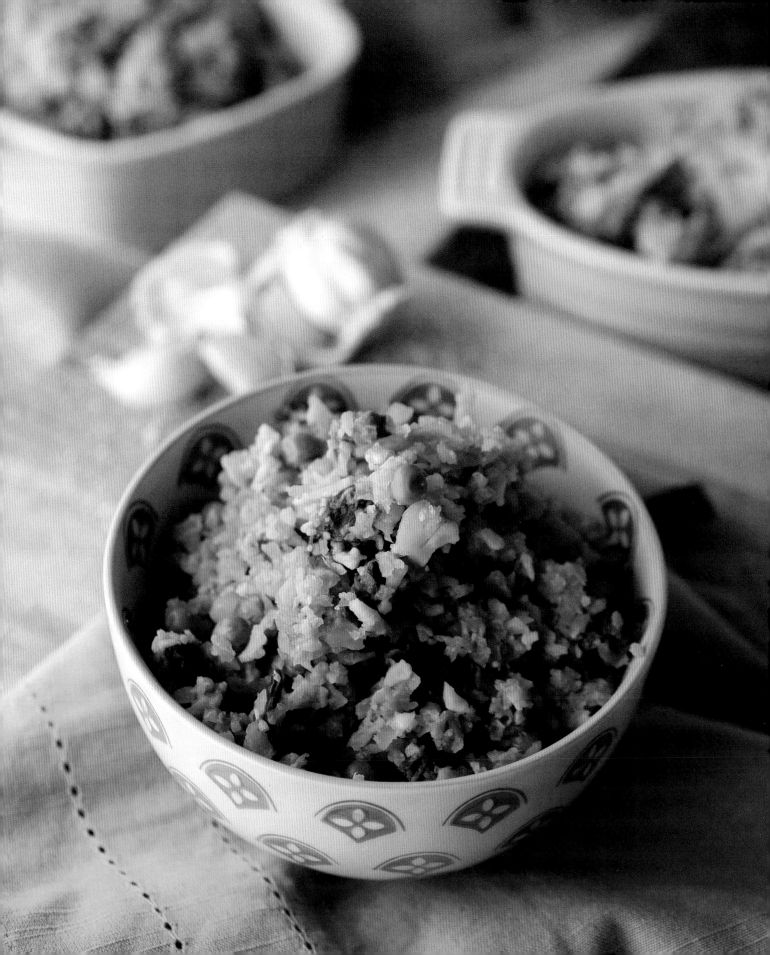

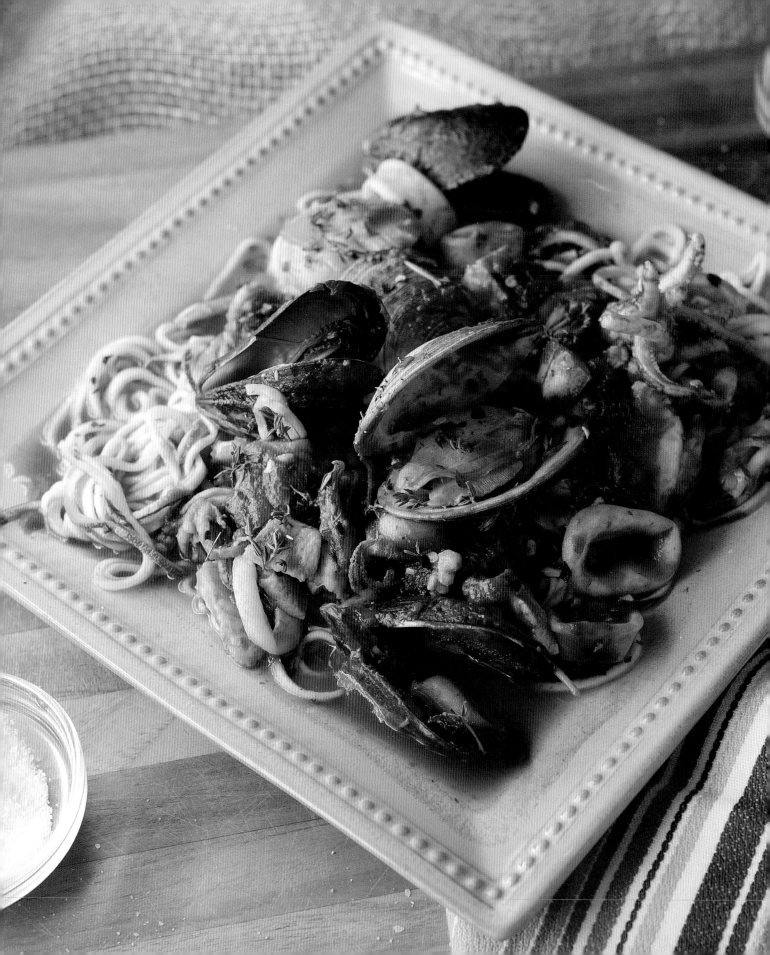

ITALIAN SEAFOOD "PASTA"

The combination of seafood, sauce and pasta is classically Italian. Nana always insisted on getting the freshest fish possible, and the kitchen smelled so good when she cooked it. If you like your sauce with a little extra heat, you can add some dried red pepper flakes.

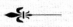 PREP TIME: 20 MINUTES
COOK TIME: 1 HOUR
SERVES: 4

¼ cup (65 ml) olive oil

1 medium onion, finely chopped

2 cloves garlic, minced

2 cups (500 ml) tomato sauce (Basic Marinara Sauce, if possible—page 29)

¾ cup (185 ml) clam or seafood broth

1 teaspoon sea salt

¾ teaspoon freshly ground black pepper

1 lb (500 g) large shrimp, shelled and deveined

1 lb (500 g) mussels, scrubbed and debearded

1 lb (500 g) clams, scrubbed

½ lb (250 g) sea scallops, muscle removed

½ lb (250 g) red snapper fillets, cut into 1½-in (3.75-cm) pieces

½ lb (250 g) small squid, cut into ½-in (1.25-cm) rings

FOR THE "PASTA"

2 large zucchinis

2 tablespoons olive oil, plus more for drizzling

1 clove garlic, minced

1 teaspoon sea salt

½ teaspoon freshly ground black pepper

½ teaspoon dried red pepper flakes

2 tablespoons chopped fresh parsley

MAKING THE SEAFOOD SAUCE

Heat a large, deep skillet or saucepan over medium heat. Add the oil and let it get very hot, then add the onion and garlic and cook until soft, about 5 minutes. Stir in the tomato sauce and clam broth and bring to a simmer.

Add the shrimp, mussels and clams and cook, uncovered, until the shells are just beginning to open and the shrimp start to curl, about 2 minutes.

Add the scallops and snapper and cook until the shells are nearly all open and the fish is nearly cooked through, 2 to 3 minutes longer. Add the squid and cook until opaque, about 1 minute.

MAKING THE ZUCCHINI "PASTA"

Cut the zucchini into very thin strips using a Spiralizer, vegetable peeler or food processor attachment.

Heat the olive oil in a skillet over medium-high heat. Add the garlic, salt, pepper, zucchini and red pepper flakes and stir-fry for about 3 minutes. Stir in the parsley, then transfer the "pasta" to a platter or large bowl.

To serve, ladle the seafood sauce over the "pasta," then drizzle with extra-virgin olive oil and top with fresh parsley.

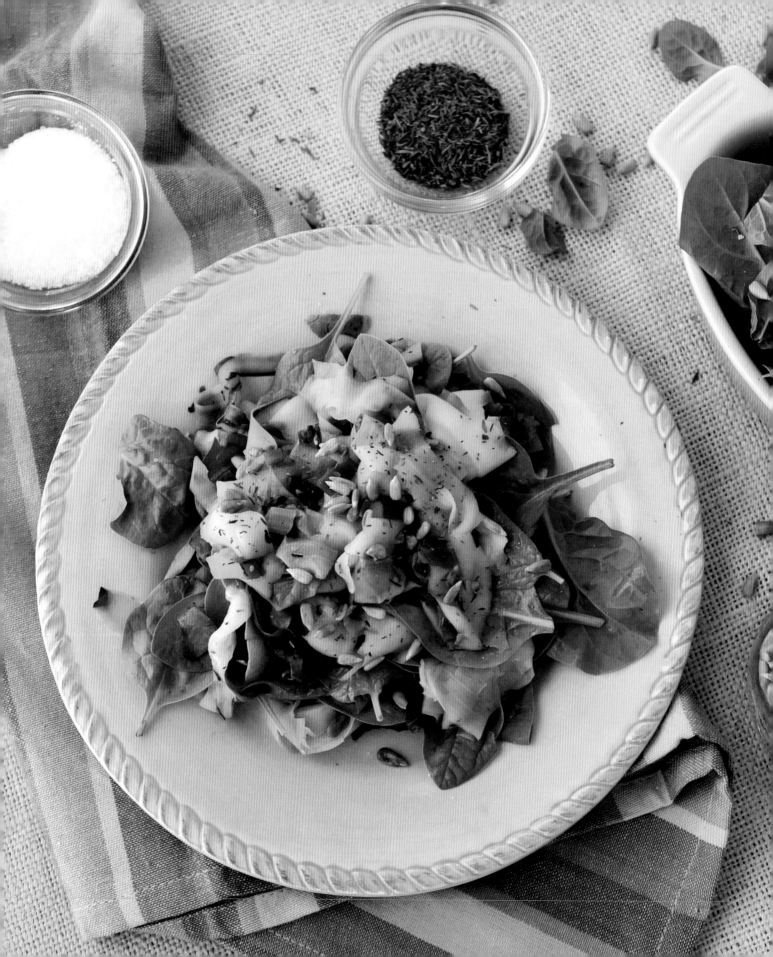

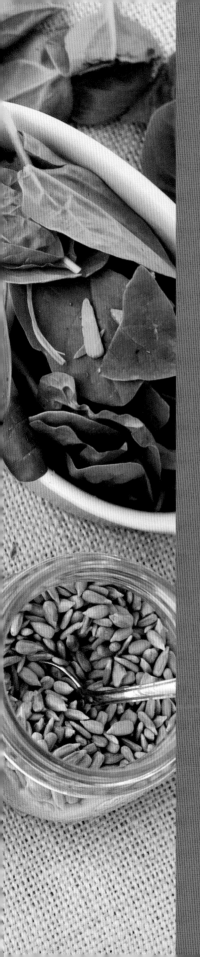

SIDE DISHES

Side dishes are anything but incidental in Italian cuisine. The sides always complement the main course, and every dish has a story that goes with it. The recipes in this section include my favorites from among those I used to make with my Nana, as well as dishes my husband and I have enjoyed during our trips to Italy. Use the freshest seasonal vegetables and herbs you can find, and don't be shy about adding tomato sauce, pancetta, or peas whenever you think they would make a good addition. Many of the side dishes in this chapter make a great breakfast when topped with an egg!

ROASTED VEGETABLES WITH BALSAMIC VINEGAR REDUCTION

The combination of many vegetables roasting in the oven brings a great aroma to the kitchen. The flavors mingle together, and the edges brown and get a little crunchy. The sweet tang of the balsamic glaze elevates the dish beyond the ordinary.

 PREP TIME: 20 MINUTES
COOK TIME: 55 MINUTES
SERVES: 4

1½ cups (375 ml) aged balsamic vinegar

2 tablespoons raw organic honey

3 carrots, sliced lengthwise, then quartered

2 large red onions, quartered

2 zucchinis, sliced lengthwise, then quartered crosswise

2 summer squash, sliced lengthwise, then sliced or quartered

1 eggplant, sliced into rounds about ¼ in (6.5 mm) thick

3 to 4 tablespoons olive oil

2 to 3 teaspoons sea salt

1½ teaspoons freshly ground black pepper

2 teaspoons dried Italian seasonings

1¼ teaspoons garlic powder

Combine vinegar and honey in a small saucepan over medium-low heat. Simmer for 15 to 20 minutes, or until reduced by half. Set aside.

Preheat oven to 375°F (190°C).

Line one or two large baking sheets with parchment paper.

Spread all the vegetables on a baking sheet (or sheets) in a single layer. Drizzle with olive oil, then season with the salt, pepper, Italian seasonings and garlic powder.

Roast for 35 minutes or until tender.

Take the roasted vegetables and set on a large platter and drizzle with balsamic glaze.

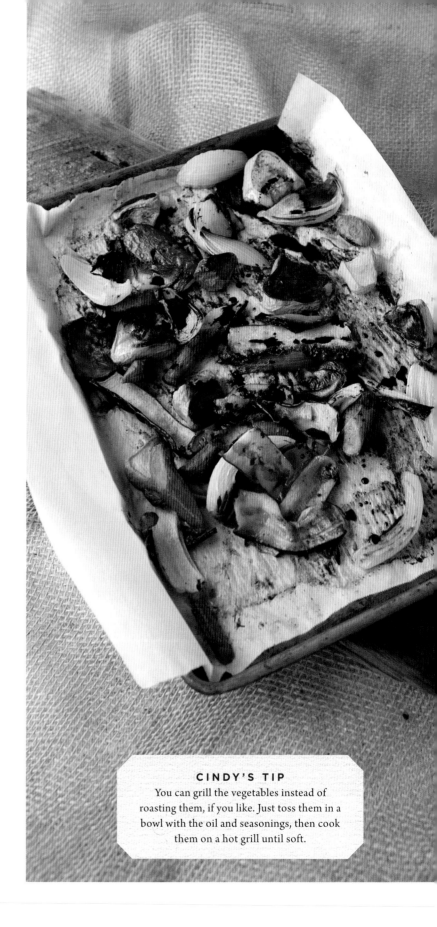

CINDY'S TIP
You can grill the vegetables instead of roasting them, if you like. Just toss them in a bowl with the oil and seasonings, then cook them on a hot grill until soft.

ROASTED CARROTS & BUTTERNUT SQUASH

This recipe was inspired by a beautiful bunch of carrots from the farmers' market and a lovely butternut squash that was sitting on my counter. I decided to slice them both into sticks and roast them. It made a wonderful side dish for a grilled steak dinner!

PREP TIME: 15 MINUTES
COOK TIME: 40 MINUTES
SERVES: 4

1 lb (500 g) butternut squash, peeled (see page 121 for peeling instructions)
1 lb (500 g) carrots, peeled
3 tablespoons olive oil
2½ teaspoons sea salt
1½ teaspoons freshly ground black pepper
2 tablespoons minced fresh chives
1 tablespoon minced fresh parsley

Preheat oven to 425°F (220°C). Line a baking sheet with parchment paper.

Cut the butternut squash in half lengthwise. Remove seeds and pulp, then slice lengthwise into ¼-in (6-mm)-thick slices. Cut slices into matchsticks.

Cut the carrots into matchsticks the same shape and thickness as the squash.

Place the squash and carrots in a large bowl. Add the olive oil, salt and pepper and toss to coat well.

Place in a single layer on the baking sheet and roast for 25 to 30 minutes, or until tender.

Add the chives and parsley and toss together, then transfer to a serving platter.

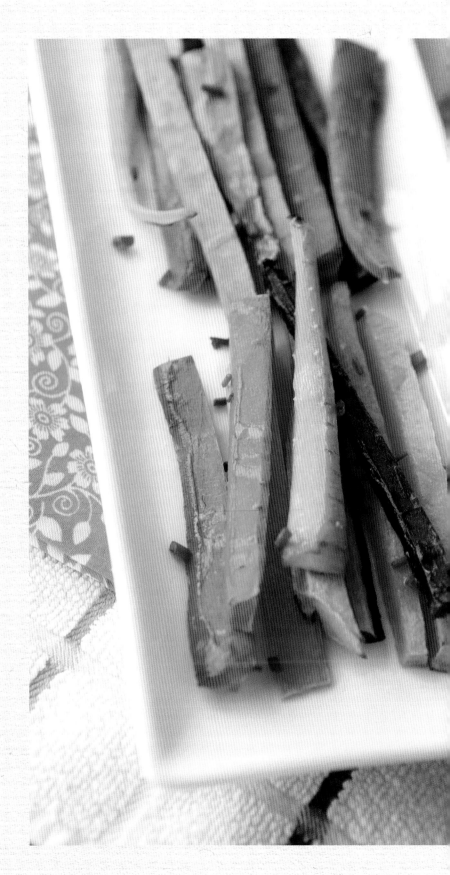

ROASTED CIPOLLINI ONIONS

Small, flat, sweet cipollini onions are a staple in Italian kitchens. Growing up, we mostly had them during the holidays, but they are great with grilled steak, burgers, and other grilled meat. Roasting makes them tender and gives them a great round, mellow flavor, which is enhanced by the balsamic vinegar. These little guys can be very addictive!

 PREP TIME: 10 MINUTES
COOK TIME: 30 MINUTES
SERVES: 4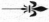

6 cups (1.5 liters) water
4 lbs (1.75 kg) cipollini onions
¾ cup (185 ml) dry red wine
¼ cup (65 ml) coconut aminos
⅓ cup (80 ml) balsamic vinegar
2 tablespoons olive oil
2 tablespoons honey
2 rosemary sprigs

Preheat oven to 425°F (220°C). Line a large baking sheet with parchment paper.

Bring water to boil in a large saucepan. Blanch the onions for 30 seconds, then remove and drain in a colander.

When the onions are cool, peel them and arrange on the baking sheet. Roast for 30 minutes.

Meanwhile, combine the wine, coconut aminos, balsamic vinegar, oil and honey in a medium saucepan over medium heat. Bring to a boil, whisking frequently, then lower the heat and simmer until it reaches a syrup-like consistency.

Place onions in a bowl and pour the glaze over, turning gently to coat. Serve in the same bowl or transfer to a serving platter. Garnish with the rosemary sprigs before serving.

CINDY'S NOTE
Coconut aminos is a soy-free seasoning which is used in many Paleo or gluten-free recipes. You will find it near the soy sauce at your local grocery store.

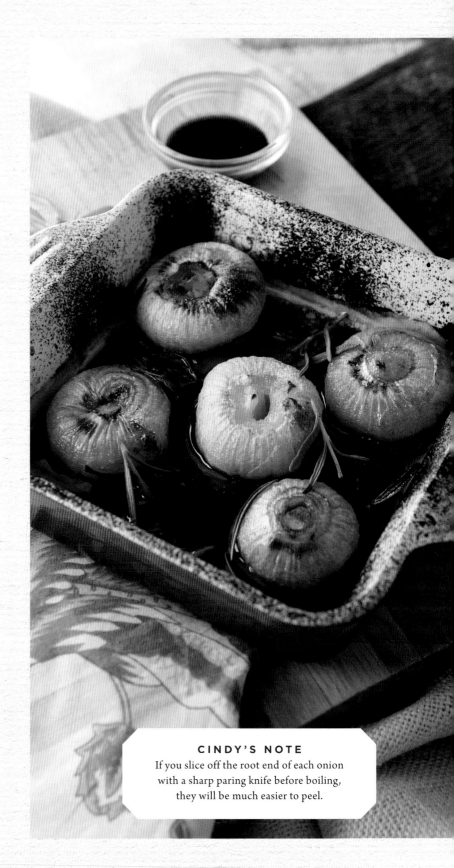

CINDY'S NOTE
If you slice off the root end of each onion with a sharp paring knife before boiling, they will be much easier to peel.

EGGPLANT & SAUSAGE CAPONATA

Caponata, a Sicilian dish, is usually served as an appetizer. You can dice it very small and use it as a dip with endive leaves or other vegetables, or make a chunkier preparation to accompany dishes such as grilled swordfish or roasted chicken.

 PREP TIME: 15 MINUTES
COOK TIME: 40 MINUTES
SERVES: 5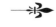

½ cup (125 ml) olive oil, divided

1 lb (500 g) pork or chicken sausage, casings removed

1 large eggplants chopped (about 4 cups / 450 g)

1 large zucchini, chopped (about 1¼ cups / 375 g)

1 large yellow onion, chopped

3 cloves garlic, minced

3 teaspoons sea salt

1 teaspoon freshly ground black pepper

One 15-oz (425-g) can crushed tomatoes

One 7-oz (200-g) can tomato paste

¼ cup (65 ml) red wine vinegar

¼ cup (35 g) capers, drained

1 cup (30 g) packed parsley leaves

1 teaspoon dried red pepper flakes

Heat a large Dutch oven over medium-high heat. Add about 2 tablespoons of the olive oil. Add the sausage and cook for about 7 minutes, breaking apart with a wooden spoon as it cooks.

Add the eggplant, zucchini, onion and garlic. Drizzle in another 2 to 3 tablespoons of olive oil, then season with the sea salt and pepper. Stir the mixture gently.

Reduce heat to medium and cook for another 7 minutes, then add the crushed tomatoes, tomato paste and red wine vinegar. Reduce heat to medium-low and cook for about 20 minutes, stirring occasionally.

Stir in the capers, parsley and red pepper flakes. Cook for another 5 minutes, or until the eggplant is golden brown and soft.

Remove from heat and enjoy!

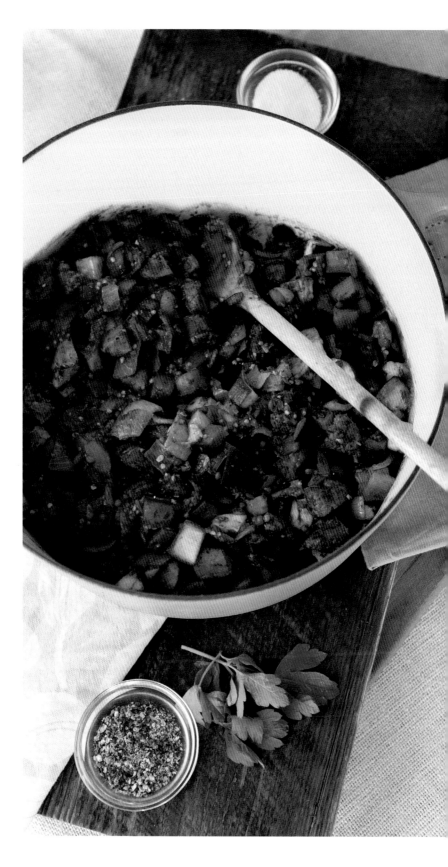

SAUTÉED ZUCCHINI RIBBONS WITH SPINACH

This dish is an excellent accompaniment to fresh grilled fish. Zucchini is amazingly versatile—it can be grilled, baked, fried, sautéed, or eaten raw in a salad. I grew up eating zucchini and eggs for breakfast. Using it in place of pasta is yet another way to enjoy this vegetable!

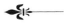

PREP TIME: 15 MINUTES
COOK TIME: 15 MINUTES
SERVES: 4

1 medium zucchini
2 to 3 tablespoons olive oil or coconut oil
2 cloves garlic, minced
3 cups (90 g) fresh baby spinach
½ cup (5 g) fresh basil, thinly sliced
2 tablespoons sunflower seeds
1 teaspoon sea salt
½ teaspoon freshly ground black pepper
Extra-virgin olive oil, for drizzling

Use a peeler or mandoline to shave ribbons from the length of the zucchini until you reach the seeds.

Heat a large skillet over medium heat and add the oil. Once hot, add the zucchini ribbons and garlic. Using tongs, toss the zucchini for 30 seconds to coat with oil and garlic.

Add the spinach and cook for about 2 minutes.

Add the basil, sunflower seeds, salt and pepper; cook for another 2 minutes.

Transfer to a large serving platter and drizzle with a little extra-virgin olive oil before serving.

CINDY'S TIP

A mandoline is very convenient for creating ribbons, but a vegetable peeler works almost as well. You may want to discard the first few strips that are just the green skin of the zucchini.

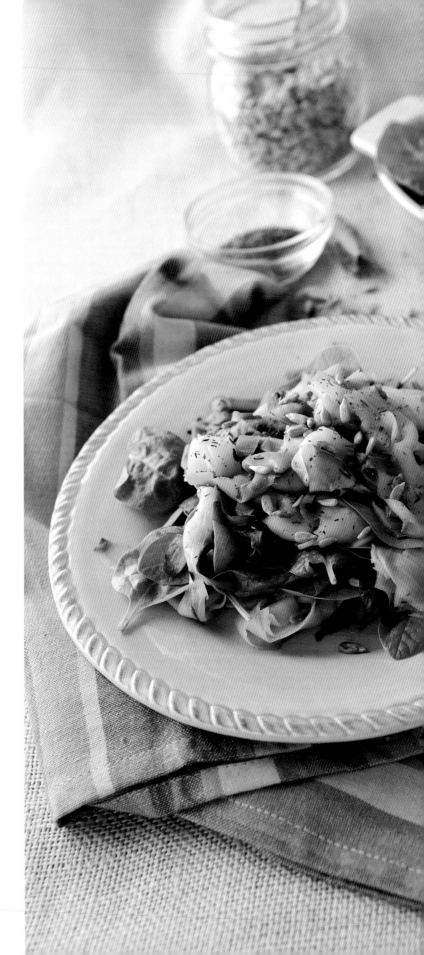

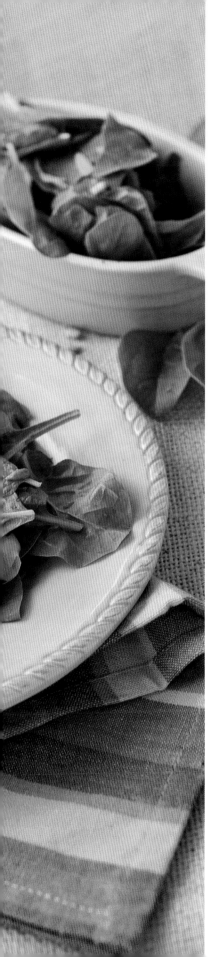

ARTICHOKES IN LEMON & HERB SAUCE

In our family, steamed artichokes were a special Sunday before-dinner treat. I have such fond memories of all of us sitting around the table before dinner with a bowl heaped with artichokes, enjoying them while laughing and talking together. What Nana loved most was to have us all together around the table with her, so this was her way of getting that to happen. I did the same with my daughter, and now we've passed on our love of artichokes to my granddaughter as well.

I devised this recipe for a slightly different take on the standard mayonnaise or lemon butter accompaniments to artichokes. Using olive oil and lots of garlic is an equally simple—and equally delicious—approach.

PREP TIME: 10 MINUTES
COOK TIME: 35 MINUTES
SERVES: 4

4 medium artichokes
3 tablespoons olive oil
3 cloves garlic, chopped
1¼ teaspoons sea salt

FOR THE LEMON AND HERB SAUCE
Juice of 1 lemon
½ teaspoon lemon zest
1 small clove garlic, minced
2 teaspoons capers, drained
2 tablespoons minced fresh dill
2 tablespoons minced flat leaf parsley
2 tablespoons extra-virgin olive oil
½ teaspoon sea salt

CINDY'S NOTE

While the heart of the artichoke is the best part, take your time getting there. Pull off a leaf, dip the fat end in sauce, and put it between your teeth, scraping off the soft meat. The leaves get smaller and more tender toward the center of the artichoke. At the bottom is the "choke," a mass of prickly fuzz that covers the heart. Just scrape this away, then slice the heart into pieces and enjoy with more sauce! Artichokes are great for a leisurely meal with family and friends.

Use a sharp knife to slice about 1 in (2.5 cm) off the top of each artichoke. Cut off the stems, leaving a 1-in (2.5-cm) stub. Holding the stem, turn the artichoke over and smack the top hard on a wooden board. This helps to open up the artichoke.

Prepare a large pot with a steamer basket by adding about 4 in (10 cm) of water (water should only come up to the bottom of a steamer basket, not cover it). Place on high heat and insert the steamer basket into the pot.

Arrange the artichokes in the steamer basket so the tops are up, then drizzle the olive oil over them. Add the garlic, pressing garlic chunks between the leaves, then season with the sea salt.

Bring to a boil, then immediately reduce heat to a medium simmer. Cook for 25 to 35 minutes, or until the outer leaves of the artichokes can be easily pulled off.

In a medium mixing bowl, combine all lemon and herb sauce ingredients.

Remove artichokes from steamer and slice in half lengthwise. Arrange on a large serving platter with a bowl of the sauce for dipping.

HERB-STUFFED ARTICHOKES

If you'd like to make a heartier dish with artichokes, rather than simply steaming them, give this one a try! It's substantial enough to serve as a meal all on its own.

PREP TIME: 10 MINUTES
COOK TIME: 45 MINUTES
SERVES: 4

4 large artichokes
¾ cup (70 g) almond meal
¼ cup (25 g) freshly grated Parmesan cheese
  (optional)
4 tablespoon olive oil, divided
2 cloves garlic, finely chopped
2 teaspoon dried basil
1½ teaspoons dried oregano
1½ teaspoons dried rosemary
1 teaspoon dried thyme
¾ teaspoon sea salt
¼ teaspoon dried red pepper flakes

Using a sharp knife, remove the top ½ in (1.25 cm) of each artichoke, and trim the stems. Smack the head of each artichoke hard against the counter or work surface to open the leaves.

Combine the almond meal, Parmesan cheese (if using), 2 tablespoons of the olive oil, garlic, basil, oregano, rosemary, thyme, salt and red pepper flakes.

Hold each artichoke over the bowl and stuff the breading into the spaces between the leaves.

Prepare a large pot with steamer basket or rack by adding water to just below the bottom of the basket and bringing to a boil.

Place the artichokes in the steamer basket or rack and drizzle the remaining 2 tablespoons of olive oil over them.

Cover and steam over medium heat for 30 to 45 minutes, or until the leaves pull away easily. Slice each artichoke in half lengthwise and arrange on a serving platter.

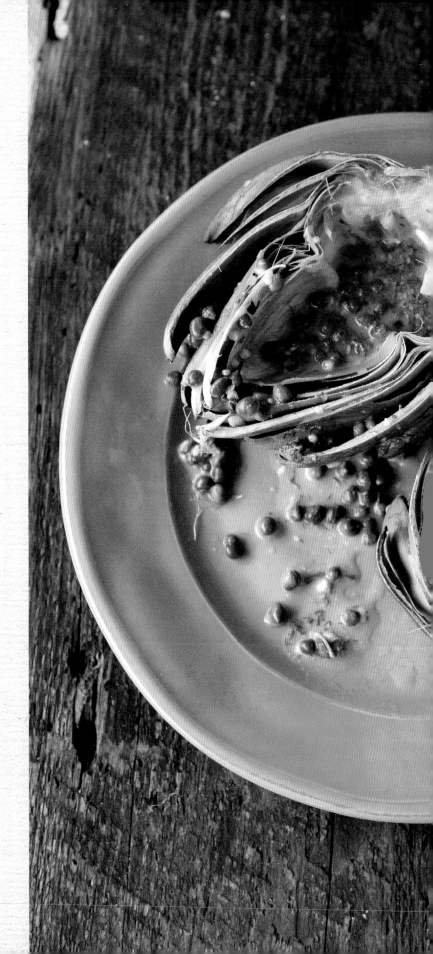

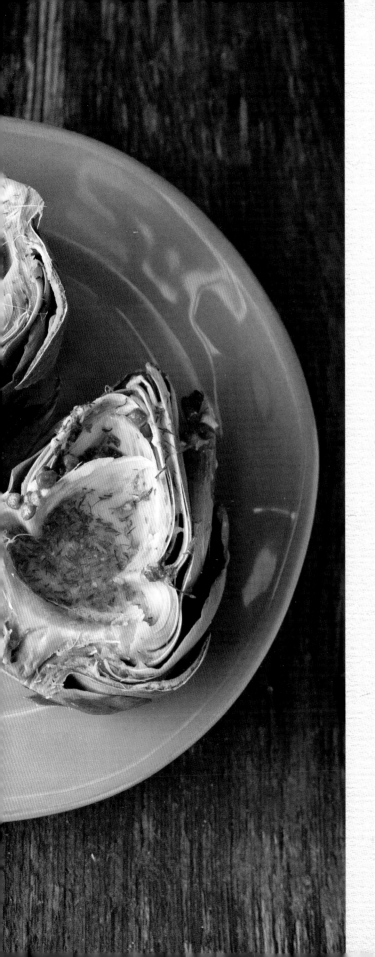

BRAISED FRESH PEAS & PANCETTA

Peas and pancetta are two things that improve any dish, Italian or otherwise! Combining them in a side dish is a sure way to make any meal special.

 PREP TIME: 10 MINUTES
COOK TIME: 15 MINUTES
SERVES: 4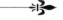

Three slices pancetta, ¼ in (6 mm) thick
1 tablespoon olive oil or coconut oil, divided
1 tablespoon unsalted butter
1 teaspoon arrowroot powder
½ cup (125 ml) chicken stock
3 green onions (scallions), green and white parts, thinly sliced
1¼ cups (150 g) green peas (fresh if possible)
1 teaspoon sea salt
½ teaspoon freshly ground black pepper
¼ teaspoon dried red pepper flakes
Juice of 1 lemon
Extra-virgin olive oil, for drizzling

Cut the pancetta into cubes.

Heat about ½ tablespoon of the oil in a skillet over medium heat. Once hot, add the pancetta and cook until crispy, about 5 minutes. Use a slotted spoon to transfer to a paper-towel-lined plate. Set aside.

Heat the remaining oil and butter in the same pan. Add the arrowroot powder and stir with a small whisk.

Slowly add the chicken stock, whisking continuously to prevent lumps.

Stir in the green onions and peas, then add the salt, pepper and red pepper flakes.

Cover and reduce heat to low. Simmer for about 5 minutes, or until the peas are fork-tender.

Taste and adjust seasonings if necessary, then stir in the lemon juice and top with the pancetta.

Just before serving, drizzle the peas with a little extra-virgin olive oil.

CINDY'S NOTE

Fresh peas work best for this recipe. If you must use frozen, reduce the amount of stock to ¼ cup and only simmer enough to heat the ingredients through.

ZUCCHINI WITH OLIVES & SUN-DRIED TOMATOES

My grandfather's enormous garden produced an abundance of zucchini every year. In zucchini season, we ate them at every meal. I'm fond of zucchini no matter how they're prepared, but sometimes I just want them in a simple salad. This one is especially nice in late summer, when it's hot and zucchini are at their peak.

PREP TIME: 15 MINUTES
COOK TIME: 15 MINUTES
SERVES: 4

2 large zucchinis

1 tablespoon chopped fresh rosemary, chopped

2 cloves garlic, minced

2 to 3 tablespoons olive oil

3 cups (120 g) chopped romaine lettuce, chopped

1 cup (30 g) baby arugula (rocket)

½ cup (120 g) olives

½ cup (120 g) sun-dried tomatoes in olive oil, chopped or sliced

4 oz (100 g) goat cheese, crumbled

Juice of 1 lemon (about 1 tablespoon)

1 teaspoon sea salt

½ teaspoon freshly ground black pepper

2 tablespoons or more extra-virgin olive oil

Cut the zucchini lengthwise to make long slices.

In a large bowl, combine the rosemary, garlic and olive oil. Add the zucchini slices and use your hands to toss them gently so they are evenly coated with the oil mixture.

Preheat an outdoor grill or indoor grill pan to medium-high.

Grill the zucchini slices for 3 to 4 minutes on each side. Set aside to cool, then cut crosswise into thirds.

Spread a layer of romaine over the bottom of a large bowl or platter, followed by the baby arugula. Add the olives and sun-dried tomatoes, then the zucchini slices. Top with crumbled goat cheese. Sprinkle the lemon juice, salt and pepper over all.

Before serving, drizzle the extra-virgin olive oil over the salad.

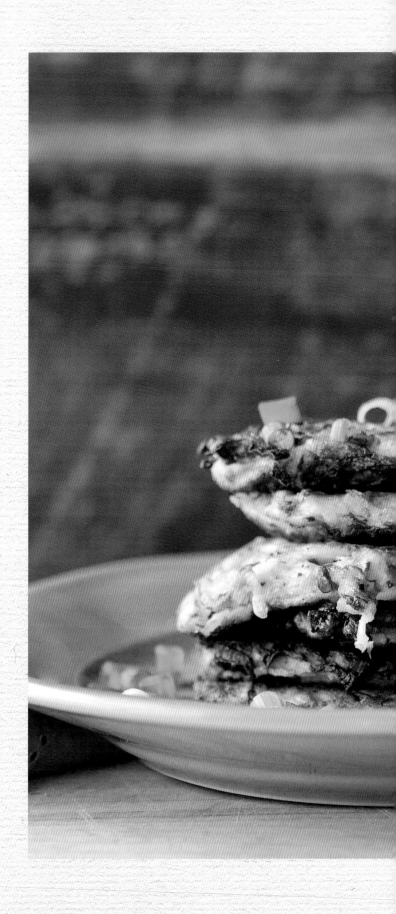

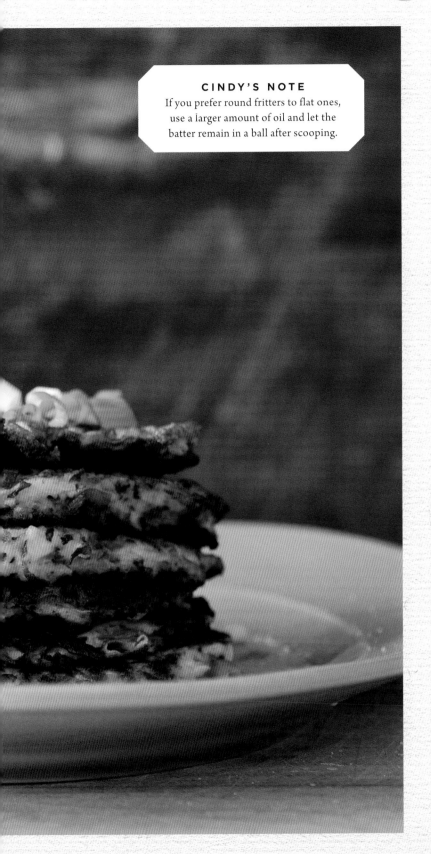

CINDY'S NOTE
If you prefer round fritters to flat ones,
use a larger amount of oil and let the
batter remain in a ball after scooping.

ZUCCHINI FRITTERS

*There's something about these zucchini fritters that
makes everyone happy! I often cook up a double batch
and freeze the extras. They're a great side dish, but
they're also wonderful for breakfast. Just warm a
leftover fritter in the microwave for 50 seconds and top
it with a poached egg.*

*You can also substitute or add other vegetables like
sweet potato, yellow onion or red bell pepper. This
is a great way to use up leftover vegetables in your
refrigerator.*

PREP TIME: 20 MINUTES
COOK TIME: 35 TO 40 MINUTES
SERVES: 4

4 small (or 2 medium) zucchinis
2 teaspoons sea salt
¼ cup (5 g) finely chopped fresh basil
¼ cup (5 g) finely chopped fresh parsley
1 teaspoon freshly ground black pepper
4 green onions (scallions), green and white parts,
 finely chopped
3 large eggs, beaten
3 tablespoons coconut flour
4 tablespoons (or more) coconut oil, for frying

Grate the zucchini on a box grater or using the grater disk
of a food processor. Place the grated zucchini in a colander
and sprinkle with salt. Let stand at least 15 minutes, then
squeeze out the resulting liquid.

Place the grated zucchini in a large mixing bowl and add
the basil, parsley, pepper, green onions, eggs and coconut
flour. Stir to combine all ingredients well. If batter is too
runny, add a little more coconut flour.

Heat the coconut oil in a large skillet or braising pan.
It is hot enough to use for frying if a drop of water sizzles
on contact.

Using an ice cream scoop to ensure that all the fritters
will be uniform, scoop batter into the hot oil and flatten
with the back of a spoon to form a fritter.

Fry until golden brown on both sides, about 2 or 3
minutes. Cook in batches so as not to overcrowd the pan.

Place the cooked fritters on a paper-towel-lined plate.
Serve warm.

VENETIAN POTATOES

When we were in Venice we had this side dish with many of our meals. It's also called patate stufate *(stewed potatoes). Like many Italian dishes, it's cooked for a long time in a large pot, which allows all the flavors to mingle.*

My Nana used to make this with her Italian pork on Saturday night, then use the leftovers in a baked egg frittata for Sunday brunch after church.

PREP TIME: 15 MINUTES
COOK TIME: 25 MINUTES
SERVES: 5

¼ cup (65 ml) olive oil
2 lbs (1 kg) of white and yellow sweet potatoes, peeled and cut into 1-in (2.5-cm) pieces
1½ teaspoons sea salt
1 teaspoon freshly ground black pepper
4 large cloves garlic, minced
One 28-oz (800-g) can diced tomatoes in juice

Heat the olive oil in a large, heavy pot over medium-high heat. Add the sweet potatoes, salt, pepper and garlic. Cook, stirring occasionally, until the potatoes begin to soften and start to stick to the bottom of the pot, about 10 minutes.

Add the diced tomatoes, then fill the can halfway with water and pour in the pot. Cover and reduce heat to medium. Continue to cook for about 20 minutes.

Using a fork, mash some of the potatoes and leave some intact. Taste and adjust seasonings if necessary.

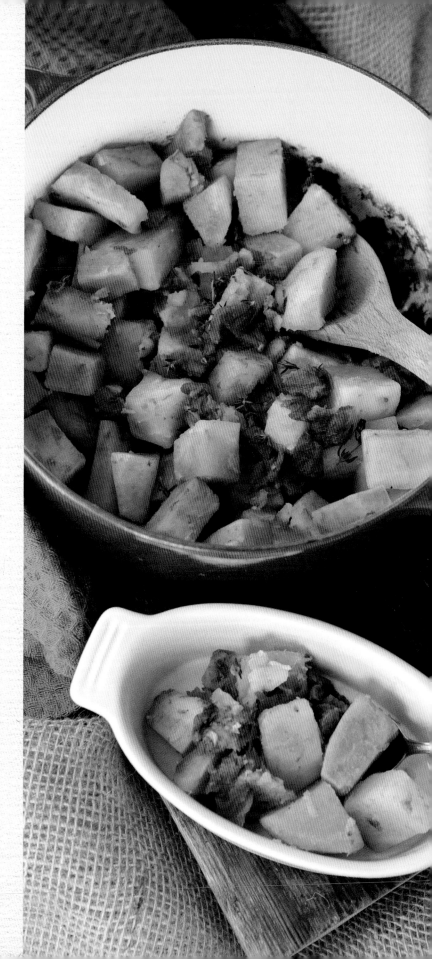

CREAMY GARLIC CAULIFLOWER "RICE"

My family loves this dish, which I serve on holidays and special occasions, but they don't realize they're eating cauliflower. I use extra garlic and, since we're Italian, add freshly grated Parmesan cheese, but you can certainly omit the cheese if you wish!

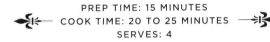

PREP TIME: 15 MINUTES
COOK TIME: 20 TO 25 MINUTES
SERVES: 4

1 head cauliflower, cut into florets

3 tablespoons olive oil

4 cloves garlic, minced

1½ teaspoons sea salt

¾ teaspoon freshly ground black pepper

¾ cup (185 ml) low-sodium chicken broth

4 tablespoons unsalted butter or ghee

¼ cup (65 ml) coconut cream or heavy cream

¼ cup (25 g) freshly grated Parmesan cheese (optional)

Fresh parsley, for garnish

Using a box grater or the grater disk of a food processor, shred the cauliflower florets to make them the size and shape of rice grains.

Heat a Dutch oven over medium heat, then add the olive oil.

When hot, add the cauliflower, garlic, salt, and pepper. Cook for 3 minutes, stirring gently with a wooden spoon. Stir in the chicken broth and cover.

Reduce the heat to medium-low and continue to cook for 12 minutes, gently stirring occasionally.

Remove the lid and add the butter and cream. Cook for another 5 minutes, stirring occasionally, so that some of the liquid is absorbed.

Once the "rice" has thickened, fold in the parsley and Parmesan cheese, if using.

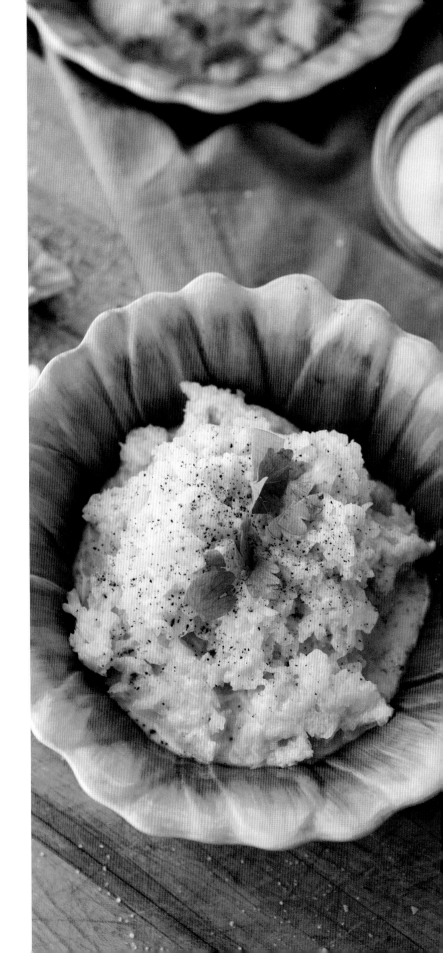

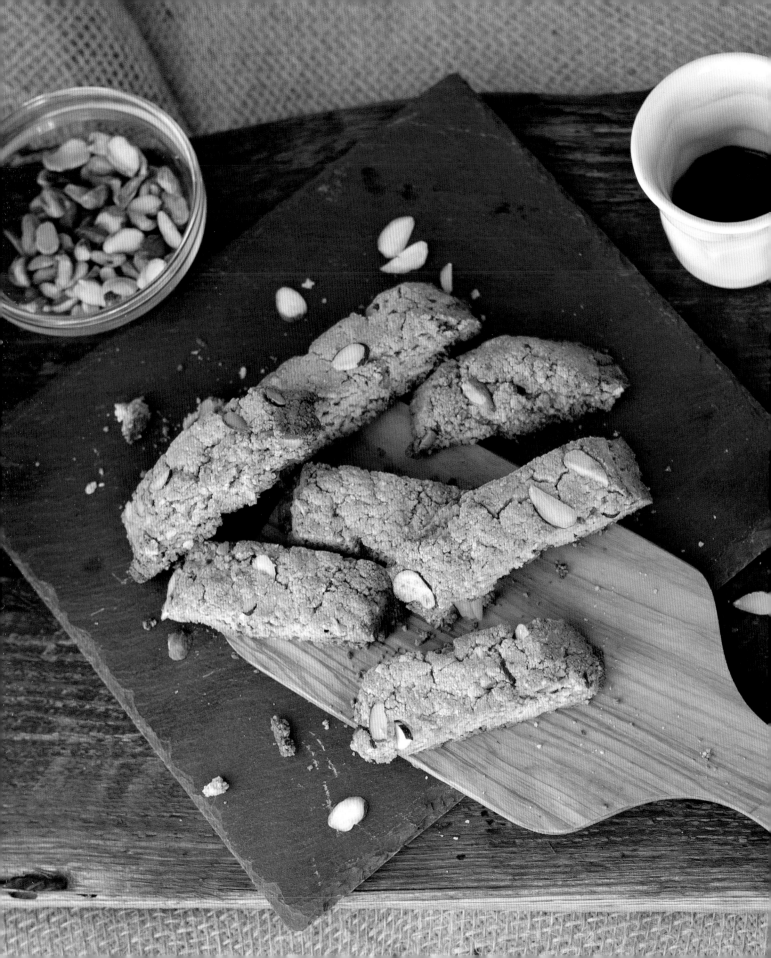

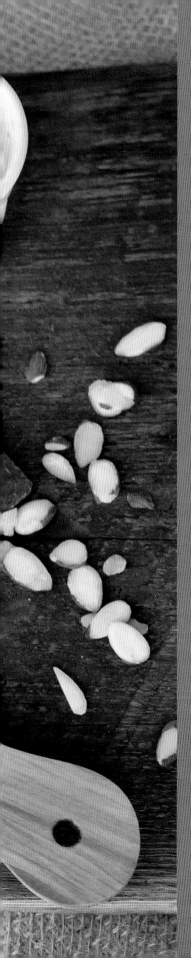

DESSERTS

A cup of espresso and a pleasurable dessert is an ideal way to end an Italian meal enjoyed with your family and friends. When we were growing up, dessert was always served in a different, smaller room. Looking back, I realize that this allowed the men and women to gather separately and chat in confidence. Nana loved being with the girls, and I am glad we had that time together.

My desserts, which are fairly simple, can be enjoyed after dinner or in the afternoon following a late lunch. Since Italians traditionally eat dinner later in the evening, they often have a light dessert after lunch. The desserts in this chapter all evoke memories of my childhood, even though they accommodate the Paleo lifestyle. I am proud to share these healthy and delectable desserts that I've created.

LEMON-RASPBERRY MERINGUE COOKIES

These pretty cookies make a dessert tray very inviting. The meringue melts in the mouth and the flavors are refreshing without being overpowering. You can get as creative as you like with these—try making different shapes and sizes, and use different kinds of fruit jam.

 PREP TIME: 10 MINUTES
COOK TIME: 2 HOURS
MAKES: 12 COOKIES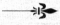

2 large egg whites, at room temperature
⅓ cup (70 g) coconut sugar
2 to 3 tablespoons all-natural seedless red raspberry jam
Juice of 1 lemon (about 1 tablespoon)

Preheat oven to 300°F (150°C). Line two baking sheets with parchment paper.

In a medium mixing bowl, use a hand mixer or eggbeater to beat egg whites until soft peaks form. Add the coconut sugar and continue beating on medium speed for 5 to 6 minutes.

Combine the jam and lemon juice in a small bowl.

Form the meringues by scooping out mounds or piping the batter from a pastry bag. Make a depression at the center of each meringue.

Bake for 2 hours, then transfer to a rack. When cool, place a teaspoonful of jam into the center of each meringue.

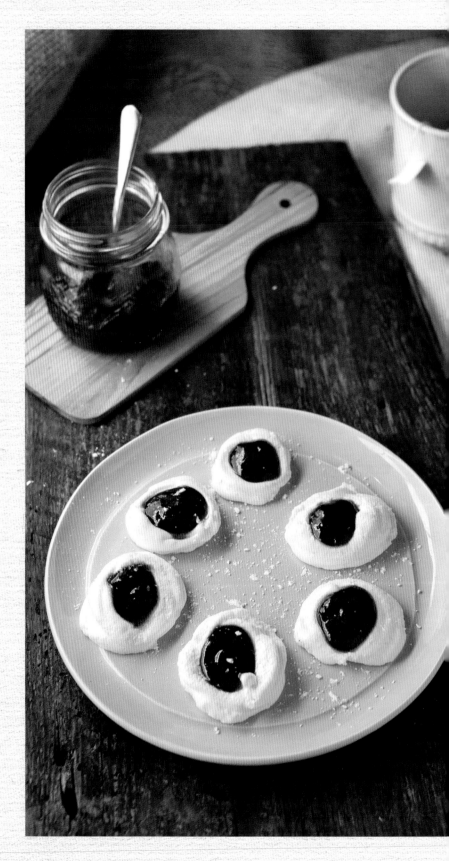

CUSTARD PIE WITH PINE NUTS & ALMONDS

Here's another great custard recipe! This one incorporates a crunchy crust that beautifully offsets the smooth, rich filling. Studded with toasted pine nuts and sliced almonds, this pie makes an impressive offering for a dinner party or special occasion.

 PREP TIME: 20 MINUTES, PLUS AT
LEAST 3 HOURS FOR REFRIGERATING
COOK TIME: 35 MINUTES
SERVES: 6

FOR THE TART CRUST

2 cups (200 g) blanched almond flour

½ teaspoon sea salt

2 tablespoons melted coconut oil, plus more for
  brushing pan

1 large egg, at room temperature

FOR THE CUSTARD FILLING

⅔ cup (135 g) coconut sugar

2 cups (475 ml) full-fat canned coconut milk

4 large egg yolks

1 vanilla bean

2 tablespoons arrowroot powder

¼ cup (30 g) sliced almonds

¼ cup (35 g) pine nuts

MAKING THE CRUST

Preheat oven to 350°F (175°C).

Combine the almond flour and salt in a food processor and pulse briefly to blend.

Add the coconut oil and egg, then continue to pulse until the dough forms a ball.

Brush a 9-in (23-cm)-diameter metal tart pan with coconut oil.

Press the dough into the pan, spreading it over the bottom and up the sides, to form the crust.

Bake for 15 minutes, then remove from oven and let cool.

PREPARING THE CUSTARD FILLING

In a saucepan over medium heat, whisk together the coconut sugar, coconut milk and egg yolks until frothy, about 5 minutes.

Split open the vanilla bean pod and scrape the inside (see page 146 for detailed instructions), then add the resulting pulp to the pan. Bring to a high simmer.

Add the arrowroot powder gradually, whisking until it is incorporated.

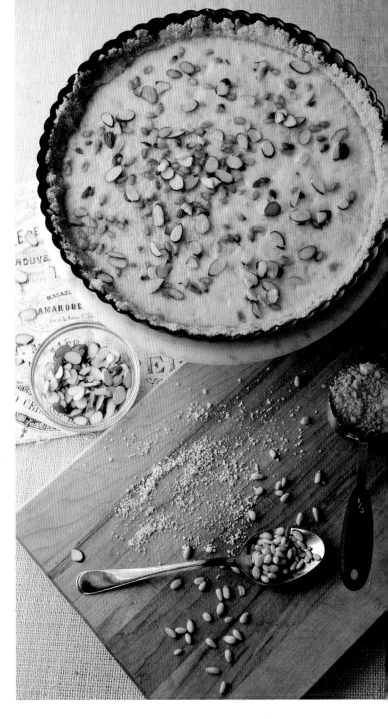

Simmer, whisking often, for about 5 minutes until mixture thickens.

Remove from heat and cover with plastic wrap. Place the wrap directly on the surface of the custard to prevent a skin from forming. Allow to cool for 30 minutes.

Meanwhile, combine the pine nuts and sliced almonds in a dry skillet and place over medium heat. Toast, shaking the pan frequently to prevent burning, until fragrant, about 2 minutes.

Pour the custard into the cooled crust and scatter the toasted nuts on top. Refrigerate for 3 hours before serving.

CREAMY COCONUT CUSTARD

Custards are my favorite desserts. In my family we always had some sort of custard and a chocolate dessert on Sundays. Most of my siblings and cousins would go for the chocolate, but Nana and I always had the custard.

This coconut custard is smooth, creamy, and satisfying—rich-tasting without being too filling. Using a real vanilla bean instead of vanilla extract adds a touch of decadence!

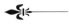

PREP TIME: 10 MINUTES
COOK TIME: 25 MINUTES
SERVES: 6

4 large eggs, at room temperature
One 13½-oz (400-ml) can full-fat coconut milk
¼ cup (55 g) coconut sugar
Pulp extracted from 1 vanilla bean (see note below)
1 teaspoon cinnamon
¼ teaspoon freshly grated nutmeg

Preheat oven to 350°F (175°C). Set a kettle of water to boil.

Whisk the eggs in a medium mixing bowl.

Heat the coconut milk in a medium saucepan over low heat. Once warm, whisk in the coconut sugar until dissolved. Add the vanilla pulp (see note below), cinnamon and nutmeg. Then pour in the eggs, whisking vigorously until blended in completely.

Place 6 ramekins or mugs in a roasting pan, making sure they are not touching each other.

Divide the custard mixture among the ramekins or mugs, then place in the oven, sliding out the rack first to minimize the possibility of spills.

Carefully pour boiling water into the roasting pan, filling it three-quarters of the way up the outside of the ramekins or mugs.

Bake for about 25 minutes. Remove from the water bath and chill in the refrigerator before serving.

EXTRACTING PULP FROM A VANILLA BEAN

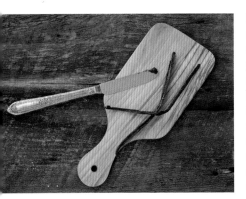

Place a vanilla bean pod on a cutting board. With a sharp paring knife, slice the pod lengthwise and split down the center. Slide the back of the knife along the inside of each half, scraping out the seeds and pulp. You can reserve the scraped pod and add it to a jar of sugar or steep in alcohol to impart a delicate vanilla flavor.

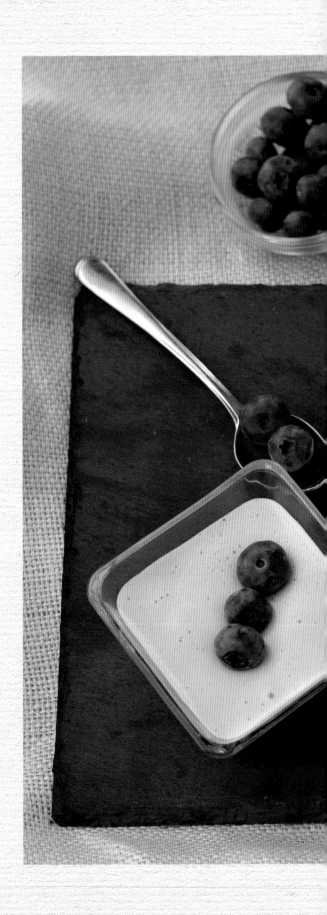

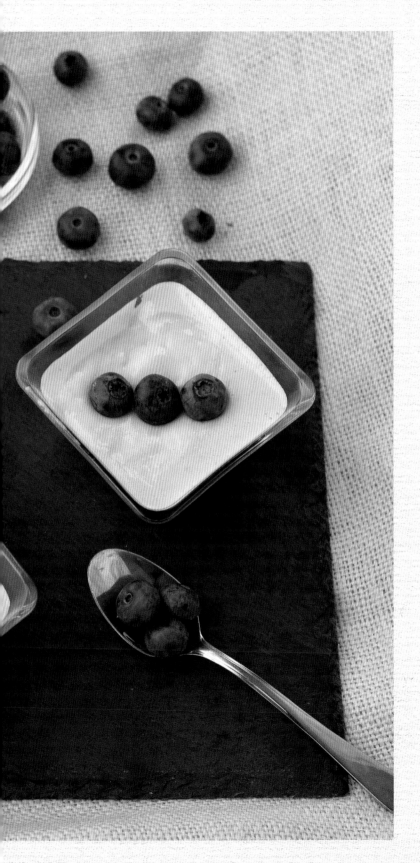

PANNA COTTA WITH BERRIES

Panna Cotta means "cooked cream" in Italian, and this delightfully rich dessert is pretty much exactly that. If you're entertaining, you can spoon the custard into wine or martini glasses the day before and keep them in the refrigerator. Just leave the berries off until you're ready to serve.

 PREP TIME: 30 MINUTES,
PLUS 3 TO 5 HOURS TO SET
COOK TIME: 15 MINUTES
SERVES: 6

1½ cups (375 ml) full-fat canned coconut milk, at room temperature
1 tablespoon unflavored powdered gelatin
2½ cups (625 ml) heavy cream
⅓ cup (80 ml) raw honey, preferably local
1 tablespoon coconut sugar
½ teaspoon vanilla extract
¼ teaspoon sea salt
2 cups (250 g) fresh berries

Pour the coconut milk into a bowl and sprinkle the gelatin over. Let stand for 5 minutes.

Transfer to a saucepan over medium heat. Stir constantly until the gelatin has dissolved and the coconut milk is hot, about 5 minutes. Do not allow the mixture to boil.

Whisk in the cream, honey, coconut sugar, vanilla and salt.

Continue whisking until the sugar has dissolved, about 5 minutes.

Remove from the heat and pour into 6 decorative glasses or mugs. Allow to cool slightly, then refrigerate until set, at least 3 hours.

Spoon berries on top before serving.

LEMON, APPLE & CARAMEL BREAD PUDDING

Bread pudding is another dessert beloved by Italians. This version, with its combination of fruit and caramel, is a comforting treat at the end of a family meal. Served alone, the lemon bread is a great accompaniment to fresh fruit or afternoon tea.

*   This is the longest recipe in the book, but it isn't complicated. Just take it one step at a time—the results are definitely worth the effort!*

PREP TIME: 30 TO 35 MINUTES
COOK TIME: 45 MINUTES
SERVES: 6

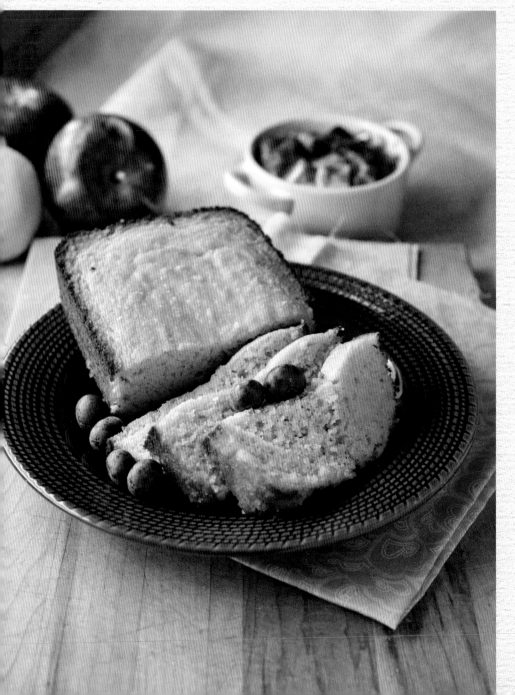

FOR THE LEMON BREAD
1½ cups (145 g) almond flour
¼ cup (30 g) coconut flour
⅓ cup (80 g) coconut sugar
1 teaspoon baking soda
1 teaspoon baking powder
½ teaspoon sea salt
Zest of 2 lemons
3 large eggs, beaten
Juice of 2 lemons
1½ teaspoons vanilla extract
⅓ cup (80 ml) full-fat canned coconut milk
3 tablespoons coconut oil, melted, plus more for brushing pan

FOR THE BREAD PUDDING
1 cup (250 ml) full-fat canned coconut milk
1 cup (250 ml) heavy cream
2 tablespoons unsalted butter
⅔ cup (135 g) coconut sugar
3 large eggs, at room temperature
1½ teaspoons cinnamon
1 teaspoon vanilla extract
¼ teaspoon freshly grated nutmeg
½ loaf Lemon Bread, cut into 1-in (2.5-cm) cubes

FOR THE APPLE TOPPING
3 baking apples, cored, peeled and chopped
Juice of 1 lemon (about 1 tablespoon)
1 teaspoon ground cinnamon
½ cup (110 g) coconut sugar
¼ cup (55 g) unsalted butter, cubed
¼ cup (30 g) chopped walnuts (optional)

FOR THE PALEO CARAMEL SAUCE
1½ cups (75 ml) full-fat canned coconut milk
½ cup (110 g) coconut sugar
1 tablespoon unsalted butter
1½ teaspoons vanilla extract
⅛ teaspoon sea salt

MAKING THE LEMON BREAD

Preheat oven to 350°F (175°C). Brush a loaf pan with coconut oil.

Combine the almond flour, coconut flour, coconut sugar, baking soda, baking powder, salt and lemon zest in a medium mixing bowl. Blend with a fork to combine and eliminate lumps.

In a separate bowl, combine the eggs, lemon juice, vanilla and coconut oil. Whisk well to blend.

Fold the wet ingredients into the dry and stir well to combine.

Turn the batter into the prepared loaf pan. Bake for 35 to 40 minutes, until a toothpick inserted into the center of the loaf comes out clean.

Remove from oven and allow to cool completely before removing from pan.

MAKING THE CUSTARD

In a saucepan over medium heat, combine the coconut milk, cream and butter. Bring to a low simmer, stirring constantly.

Whisk in the coconut sugar, eggs, cinnamon, nutmeg and vanilla. Continue to cook, stirring constantly, until the mixture thickens. Remove from heat.

ASSEMBLING THE PUDDING

Combine all apple topping ingredients in a mixing bowl. Stir well to combine, then set aside. Preheat oven to 350°F (175°C).

Brush 6 ramekins (for individual servings) or one baking dish (for family-style serving) with coconut oil.

Fill the ramekins or baking dish halfway with the cubed bread, then pour the custard mixture over (the vessels should not be more than three-quarters full). Top with the apples, then place the ramekins or dish on a baking sheet.

Bake for about 25 minutes.

PREPARING THE SAUCE

Combine the coconut milk and coconut sugar in a saucepan over medium heat and bring to a boil, whisking constantly. Continue to whisk gently as you add the butter, vanilla and sea salt. Reduce the heat to low and continue stirring for about 5 minutes.

Remove from heat and transfer to a bowl to cool. Whisk vigorously until glossy.

Drizzle caramel sauce over the bread pudding just before serving.

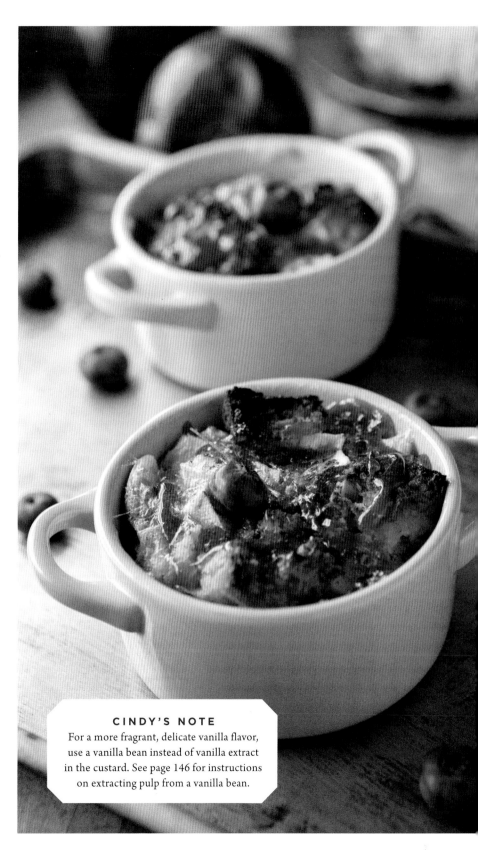

CINDY'S NOTE

For a more fragrant, delicate vanilla flavor, use a vanilla bean instead of vanilla extract in the custard. See page 146 for instructions on extracting pulp from a vanilla bean.

RASPBERRY & PISTACHIO SEMIFREDDO

Semifreddo, which means half cold or half frozen in Italian, is typically an ice cream that almost has the texture of a mousse. The flavorings in this delicate dessert can be varied according to the season and your tastes. To me, raspberries and pistachios are an ideal combination, but you can be creative with your choices.

 PREP TIME: 10 MINUTES,
PLUS AT LEAST
6 HOURS FREEZING TIME
SERVES: 6

6 large egg yolks

3 tablespoons, plus 1 teaspoon honey, plus more for drizzling

1 cup (250 ml) whipping cream

8 oz (250 g) fresh raspberries plus a few extra to serve and/or puree

2½ tablespoons chopped pistachio meats

In a medium bowl, combine egg yolks and honey using an electric mixer. Beat for about 10 minutes, or until the mixture becomes pale and creamy.

In a separate bowl, whip the heavy cream with the hand mixer until stiff, about 3 or 4 minutes. Gently fold the whipped cream into the egg mixture.

Line a loaf tin with parchment paper so that the paper hangs over the edges of the pan. Pour the mixture in and cover with the excess parchment or clear wrap.

Place in freezer for 1½ hours, or until the mixture has just begun to freeze. Then stir in the raspberries and pistachios so they are evenly distributed throughout the mixture. Re-cover with the parchment paper or clear wrap and return to the freezer until completely frozen.

Allow the semifreddo to soften in the refrigerator 15 minutes prior to serving. Turn out of the tin onto a shallow serving platter and cut into slices. Serve with extra raspberries and a drizzle of honey on each serving.

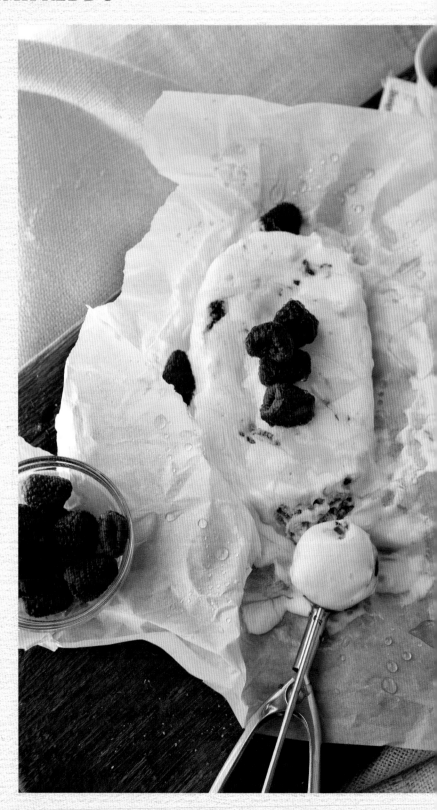

PISTACHIO & ALMOND BISCOTTI

This is the classic twice-baked "biscotti," as they are known in the United States. (In Italian, "biscotti" is just a generic word for cookies or biscuits.) The double baking makes the cookies crisp but not dry—just the thing for enjoying with an espresso.

PREP TIME: 15 MINUTES
COOK TIME: 2 HOURS
SERVES: 6

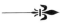

1 cup (100 g) blanched almond flour
½ cup (50 g) coconut flour
½ teaspoon baking soda
¼ teaspoon sea salt
½ cup (125 ml) maple syrup
1 teaspoon almond extract
¼ cup (30 g) sliced almonds
¼ cup (30 g) chopped pistachio meats

Preheat oven to 350°F (175°C). Line a baking sheet with parchment paper.

Combine the almond flour, coconut flour, baking soda, and salt in a food processor and pulse few times to blend.

Add the almond extract and maple syrup and process on low to make a stiff dough.

Using a rubber spatula, transfer the dough to a large bowl and stir in the almonds and pistachios.

Place the dough on the parchment-lined baking sheet. Wet your hands to keep the dough from sticking and form the dough into a log about 1 in (2.5 cm) thick.

Bake for 15 minutes, then remove from oven and let cool for about 1½ hours.

Bring the oven back up to 350°F (175°C). Cut the log into ½-in (1.25-cm)-thick slices. Arrange the slices flat on the baking sheet and return to the oven for 15 minutes.

Turn off the heat, crack open the oven door and leave the cookies there until they have cooled.

Serve cookies immediately or store in a sealed container.

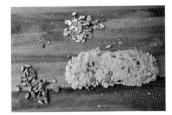

Stir the almonds and pistachios into the dough.

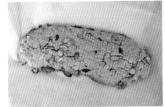

Place the dough on a parchment-lined baking sheet and form into a narrow log before baking.

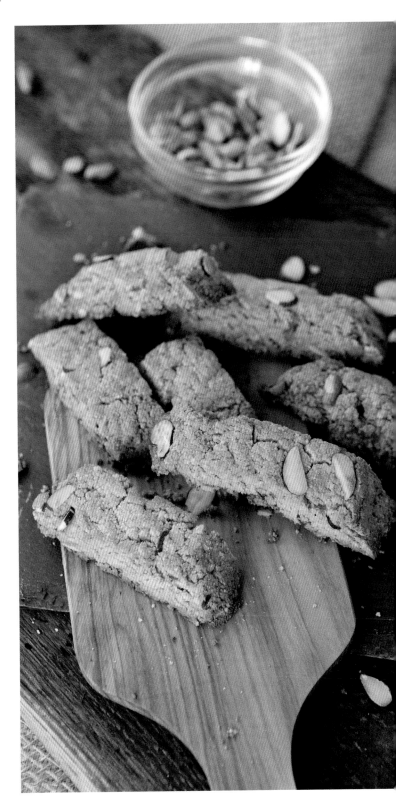

PROSECCO & PEACH COCKTAILS

Prosecco and frozen peaches can be combined to create an elegant sparkling cocktail reminiscent of a Bellini. One of my favorite things to do in Venice is to sit at an outdoor café or restaurant and enjoy a Bellini while people-watching. The costumed and masked actors who interact with tourists and entertain children are especially fun to watch.

Since discovering this cocktail, I've gotten in the habit of keeping frozen peaches and a few bottles of chilled prosecco on hand to serve as a welcome drink or to enjoy as a dessert. It's a refreshing departure from the usual white wine or sherry aperitif.

 **PREP TIME: 5 MINUTES
SERVES: 6 TO 8**

1 bottle prosecco
6 to 8 frozen peach slices slices

Prepare 6 or 8 champagne glasses or wineglasses. Place a peach slice in each one.

Pour in prosecco, and serve with a smile.

CINDY'S NOTE
You can slice up fresh peaches when in season and freeze them in a plastic resealable bag, or simply keep a bag of store-bought frozen peaches on hand. Do not allow peaches to thaw, and use within three months.

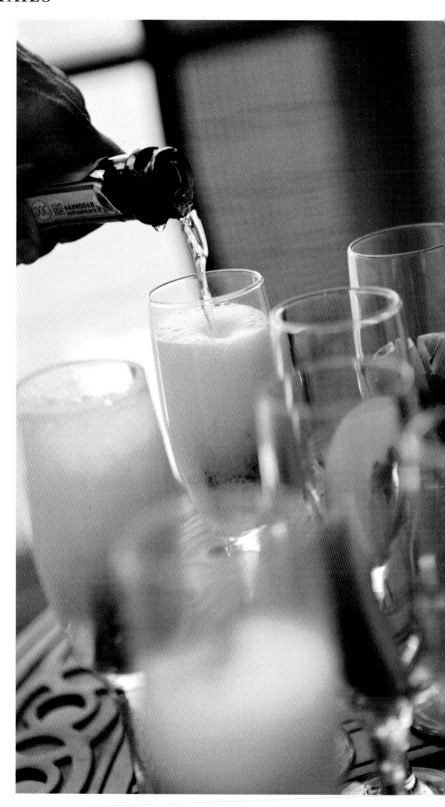

CHOCOLATE POTS DE CRÈME

In spite of its simplicity, this recipe is an enduring favorite with my family. Plus, it's fun to say "Chocolate Pots de Crème" with an exaggerated French accent!

 PREP TIME: 10 MINUTES, PLUS
2 HOURS TO REFRIGERATE
COOK TIME: 10 MINUTES
SERVES: 4

1 cup (250 ml) full-fat canned coconut milk
3 egg yolks
6 oz (170 g) ounces unsweetened dark
  chocolate, chopped
¼ cup (55 g) coconut sugar
1 teaspoon vanilla extract
⅛ teaspoon sea salt

Warm coconut milk in a saucepan over medium-low heat. Whisk in the egg yolks.

Add the chocolate, sugar, vanilla and salt, whisking continuously until the chocolate is melted.

Bring to a high simmer, but do not allow mixture to boil. Cook for 5 minutes.

Pour into 4 ramekins, distributing evenly. Cover with clear wrap, allowing the wrap to contact the surface of the pudding so a skin does not form. Refrigerate for 2 hours.

Serve accompanied by coconut cream or fresh fruit.

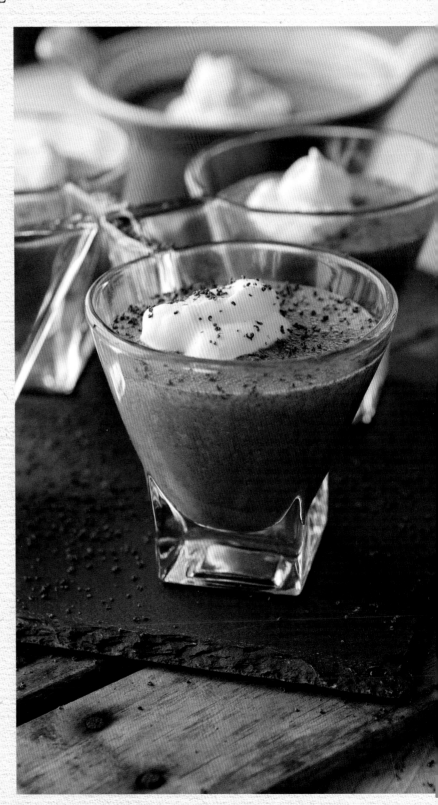

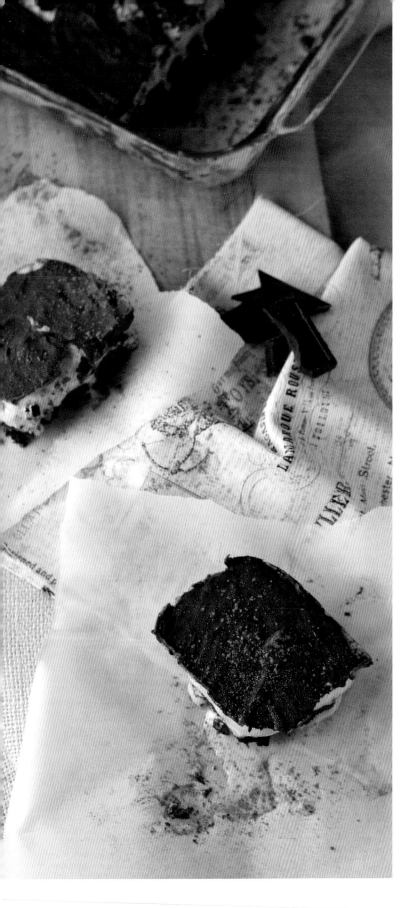

BROWNIE & COFFEE FROZEN CUSTARD SUNDAE

An Italian dessert that I am particularly fond of is chocolate ganache with coffee ice cream. It's always a special treat for me when I travel to Italy, and I wanted to adapt it to the Paleo style of eating. I modified the recipe, removing all dairy ingredients and processed sugar, and was surprised to find that the flavors were more intense and satisfying. The brownie really sates my chocolate cravings without compromising my commitment to healthier eating.

 PREP TIME: 30 MINUTES, PLUS AT
LEAST 5 HOURS FOR FREEZING
COOK TIME: 35 MINUTES
SERVES: 8 TO 10

FOR THE BROWNIES
Melted coconut oil, for brushing pan
½ cup (60 g) unsweetened cocoa powder
½ teaspoon sea salt
1 teaspoon baking soda
½ teaspoon baking powder
1 ripe banana
2 cups (480 g) almond butter
3 large eggs, at room temperature
1 teaspoon vanilla extract
1 cup (340 g) raw honey, preferably local
4 oz (115 g) unsweetened dark chocolate

FOR THE FROZEN CUSTARD
1½ cups (375 ml) canned full-fat coconut milk
2 tablespoons strong brewed coffee, cooled to room
  temperature
2 tablespoons raw honey, preferably local
2 large egg yolks
1 teaspoon vanilla extract
Freshly ground coffee beans (optional, for garnish)

FOR THE CHOCOLATE GANACHE
1¾ cups (280 g) all-natural semi-sweet chocolate chips
⅓ cup (80 ml) palm oil shortening

MAKING THE BROWNIES

Preheat oven to 350°F (175°C). Brush a glass 9 x 13-in (23 x 33-cm) pan with melted coconut oil.

Sift the cocoa powder, salt, baking soda and baking powder together into a mixing bowl and set aside.

In a small bowl, mash the banana, then whisk in the almond butter, eggs, vanilla and honey.

Place the chocolate in a microwave-safe bowl and microwave for 45 seconds, then stir with a small spoon or rubber spatula until smooth.

Fold the banana mixture into the dry ingredients, then add the melted chocolate. Combine well.

Pour the batter into the prepared glass pan and bake for 35 minutes, or until a toothpick inserted into the center comes out clean.

Let cool for 15 minutes, then place in the freezer for 1 hour.

MAKING THE FROZEN CUSTARD

Combine the coconut milk, coffee, honey, egg yolks, and vanilla in a saucepan. Place over medium heat and whisk until the mixture just begins to bubble. Immediately remove from heat and allow to cool.

Transfer the mixture to a bowl and cover with plastic wrap. Make sure the wrap touches the surface of the custard to prevent a skin from forming. Refrigerate for at least 2 hours, or overnight.

Freeze the custard in an ice cream machine, following the manufacturer's directions, until the desired consistency is reached. Prepare the sundaes immediately.

ASSEMBLE THE SUNDAES

Take the pan of brownies out of the freezer and cover with an even layer of the coffee frozen custard. Return to the freezer for 15 minutes.

Meanwhile, make the chocolate ganache by combining the chocolate chips and palm oil shortening in a small microwave-safe bowl. Microwave for 45 seconds, then whisk vigorously until the chocolate is melted.

Take the glass pan out of the freezer again and cover the frozen custard with the chocolate ganache. Freeze for another 3 or 4 hours.

Garnish with a sprinkle of ground coffee beans, if desired, and serve.

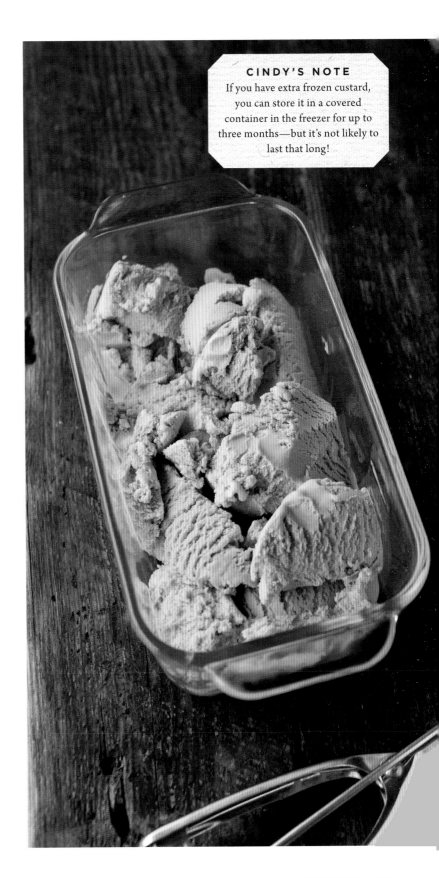

CINDY'S NOTE

If you have extra frozen custard, you can store it in a covered container in the freezer for up to three months—but it's not likely to last that long!

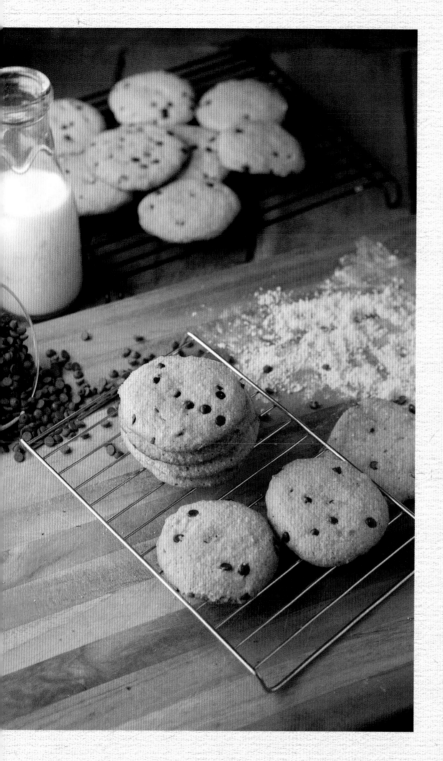

CHOCOLATE CHIP COOKIES

Sometimes you just crave your old favorites, and if it's chocolate-chip cookies you want, these are just the ticket. The first time I made them, they vanished very fast—mostly because I was eating them! Now I make them on a regular basis, but I try to be better about sharing them with others.

 PREP TIME: 15 MINUTES
COOK TIME: 14 MINUTES
MAKES: 8 COOKIES

½ cup (100 g) palm oil shortening
½ cup (125 g) coconut sugar
2 large eggs, at room temperature
1 teaspoon baking soda
½ teaspoon baking powder
¾ teaspoon sea salt
1 teaspoon vanilla extract
3 cups (290 g) almond flour
1¼ cups (200 g) chocolate chips

Preheat oven to 375°F (190°C). Line a large baking sheet with parchment paper.

In a large mixing bowl, combine the palm oil shortening and coconut sugar and cream with a wooden spoon or hand mixer. Add the eggs, baking soda, baking powder, and vanilla, and continue to mix until smooth.

Add the almond flour and mix (at medium speed if using a hand mixer) for 1 minute. Fold in the chocolate chips.

Use a tablespoon to scoop out balls of dough onto the baking sheet. Bake for 13 to 14 minutes.

Let cool on a wire rack, then transfer to a platter to serve.

CHOCOLATE ALMOND TORTE

What's not to like about a torte? The name sounds fancy, and it looks so beautiful on a cake stand. The combination of chocolate and almonds in this torte, perhaps enjoyed with a glass of red wine while sitting by the fire, makes a fantastic sweet ending to a meal.

 PREP TIME: 15 MINUTES
COOK TIME: 40 MINUTES
SERVES: 6

2 tablespoons coconut oil, melted

1½ cups (280 g) whole almonds

1 cup (220 g) coconut sugar

1 cup (180 g) unsweetened chocolate, chopped

5 large eggs, separated

¾ teaspoon almond extract

1 stick (8 tablespoons) unsalted butter,
  melted and cooled

½ teaspoon sea salt

Preheat oven to 350°F (175°C).

Brush melted coconut oil on the bottom and 2 inches (5 cm) up the sides of a 10-in (25-cm) diameter springform pan. Wrap the bottom ½ inch (1.25 cm) of the pan in foil and place on a baking sheet.

Combine the almonds and ½ cup of the coconut sugar in a food processor. Pulse until almonds are very finely ground but not uniform. Transfer to a mixing bowl.

In the same food processor, combine the chocolate and another ¼ cup of the coconut sugar. Process until the chocolate is finely ground, but do not let it begin to clump. Add to the almond mixture and combine.

Using a hand mixer, beat the egg yolks and the remaining ¼ cup coconut sugar in a mixing bowl until mixture begins to thicken, about 3 or 4 minutes. Add the almond extract and beat for another 30 seconds to combine.

Fold the chocolate-almond mixture into the egg yolks, then stir in the melted butter.

Beat the egg whites with an eggbeater or hand mixer. Add the salt and continue mixing until stiff peaks begin to form. Gently fold the whites into the chocolate batter, being careful not to overmix.

Bake for about 40 minutes, or until a toothpick comes out clean when inserted in the middle of the torte.

Transfer the pan to a rack and allow to cool completely. Set onto a serving platter or cake stand, then release the sides of the pan.

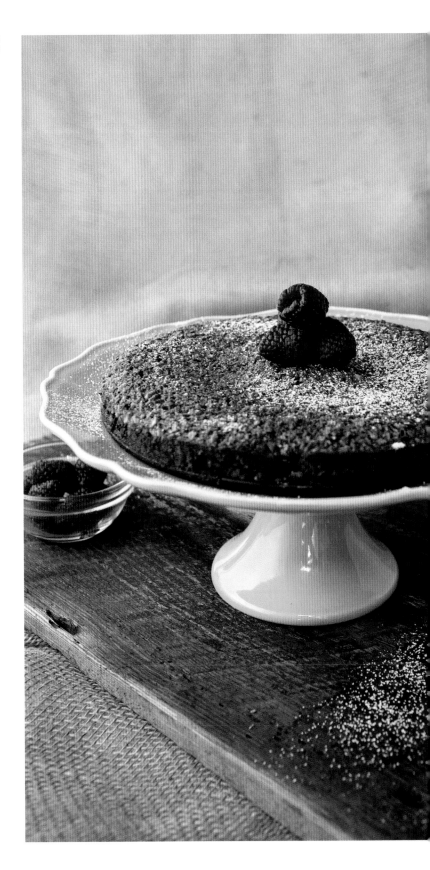

INDEX

ACKNOWLEDGMENTS

I am extremely thankful and grateful for the continued support from my friends in Connecticut. I offer my appreciation to the following amazing and caring people who have helped me so much along the way.

Jordan Coe, owner of Shop Rite (E. Hartford and Manchester), thanks for your generosity and continued support for my TV segments, non-profit demonstrations and magazine, as well as this cookbook. I appreciate the time and effort you and your team put in to help me do my shopping for *Cindy's Table.*

Danny and Rosanna D'Aprile, owners of D&D Market in Hartford, CT, I love your Italian market and all of your specialty items from Italy that make my recipes so much better. Your store brings back memories of shopping at Italian markets with Nana on Saturdays. I appreciate your continued support for my TV segments, my magazine and this cookbook!

To the amazing family of City Fish in Wethersfield, CT, you have all been so supportive. I love how Telly always chooses the best-looking fish for my photos. Your seafood is the freshest, and I am always honored to say "I got this from City Fish." Thank you for everything, including your wonderful friendship.

A special thank-you to Le Creuset, Hamilton Beach, Emily Henry, Schmidt Bros. and Bialetti, for making items that work perfectly for my style of cooking. I appreciate the confidence you have shown in me and by sending me your products to use in my TV segments, the magazine, at other events and in this cookbook.

To my friends at Venora's salon, thank you so much for making sure I was ready for my photo shoots! I'm especially grateful to Kristy, who came to my house at 7 a.m. to do my hair; and Cathy, who arrived right behind her to do my makeup. We certainly had a lot of laughs in my bathroom.

The biggest thank-you goes to my husband and kids. You have all been so patient with me when I have to take pictures before we eat our meals together. I love you all so much. Glenn, you are an amazing husband and my best friend; I am so glad to be sharing this journey with you!

Published by Tuttle Publishing, an imprint of Periplus Editions (HK) Ltd.

www.tuttlepublishing.com

Copyright © 2015 Cindy Barbieri

All rights reserved. No part of this publication may be reproduced or utilized in any form or by any means, electronic or mechanical, including photocopying, recording, or by any information storage and retrieval system, without prior written permission from the publisher.

Library of Congress Cataloging-in-Publication Data

Barbieri, Cindy, 1964-
 Paleo Italian cooking : authentic Italian gluten-free family recipes / Cindy Barbieri ; photography by Nicole Alekson.
    pages cm
 Includes index.
 ISBN 978-0-8048-4512-0 (pbk.) -- ISBN 978-1-4629-1718-1 (ebook) 1. Cooking, Italian. 2. Gluten-free diet--Recipes. 3. Low-carbohydrate diet--Recipes. 4. High-protein diet--Recipes. 5. Prehistoric peoples--Food. I. Alekson, Nicole. II. Title.
 TX723.B24168 2015
 641.5945--dc23
                    2015017492

ISBN: 978-0-8048-4512-0

PHOTO CREDITS
Dreamstime: Petr Jilek 12; Tomas Marek 10, 13; Piliphoto 97
Robb Wolf 4
Schmidt Brothers Cutlery 22 (bottom)
All other photography by Nicole Alekson
Food styling by Lindsey Frey

DISTRIBUTED BY
North America, Latin America & Europe
Tuttle Publishing
364 Innovation Drive
North Clarendon, VT 05759-9436 U.S.A.
Tel: (802) 773-8930; Fax: (802) 773-6993
info@tuttlepublishing.com
www.tuttlepublishing.com

Japan
Tuttle Publishing
Yaekari Building, 3rd Floor
5-4-12 Osaki, Shinagawa-ku
Tokyo 141 0032
Tel: (81) 3 5437-0171; Fax: (81) 3 5437-0755
sales@tuttle.co.jp; www.tuttle.co.jp

Asia Pacific
Berkeley Books Pte. Ltd.
61 Tai Seng Avenue #02-12
Singapore 534167
Tel: (65) 6280-1330; Fax: (65) 6280-6290
inquiries@periplus.com.sg; www.periplus.com

19 18 17 16 15
5 4 3 2 1

Printed in Malaysia   1507 TW

TUTTLE PUBLISHING® is a registered trademark of Tuttle Publishing, a division of Periplus Editions (HK) Ltd.

THE TUTTLE STORY
"BOOKS TO SPAN THE EAST AND WEST"

Many people are surprised to learn that the world's leading publisher of books on Asia had humble beginnings in the tiny American state of Vermont. The company's founder, Charles E. Tuttle, belonged to a New England family steeped in publishing.

Immediately after WWII, Tuttle served in Tokyo under General Douglas MacArthur and was tasked with reviving the Japanese publishing industry. He later founded the Charles E. Tuttle Publishing Company, which thrives today as one of the world's leading independent publishers.

Though a westerner, Tuttle was hugely instrumental in bringing a knowledge of Japan and Asia to a world hungry for information about the East. By the time of his death in 1993, Tuttle had published over 6,000 books on Asian culture, history and art—a legacy honored by the Japanese emperor with the "Order of the Sacred Treasure," the highest tribute Japan can bestow upon a non-Japanese.

With a backlist of 1,500 titles, Tuttle Publishing is more active today than at any time in its past—inspired by Charles Tuttle's core mission to publish fine books to span the East and West and provide a greater understanding of each.